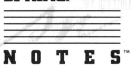

SPRING!

N O T E S™

FLUIDS AND ELECTROLYTES

Sheryl A. Innerarity, RN, PhD

Dr. Innerarity, this book's coauthor, is an Assistant Professor of Nursing at the University of Texas, Austin. She received her BA in History and ADN from Midwestern University, Wichita Falls, Tex.; her BSN and MSN from the University of Texas at Arlington; and her PhD from Texas Woman's University, Denton. Dr. Innerarity is a member of Sigma Theta Tau, the American Nurses' Association, the Texas Nurses' Association, and the Texas Association of College Teachers.

June L. Stark, RN, BSN, CCRN

Ms. Stark, this book's coauthor, is a Critical-Care Instructor and Renal Nurse Consultant for New England Medical Center Hospitals, Boston. She received her RN from Jackson Memorial School of Nursing, Miami, Fla., and her BSN from Salem (Mass.) State College. Ms. Stark is a member of the American Association of Critical-Care Nurses, the Massachusetts Nurses' Association, and the American Nephrology Nurses' Association.

Luana Martindale, RN, MSN

Ms. Martindale, this book's reviewer, is an Associate Professor of Nursing at the University of Arkansas at Little Rock. She received her BSN from the Deaconess School of Nursing, Evansville, Ind., and her BSN and MSN from the University of Evansville. Ms. Martindale is a member of the Arkansas State Nurses' Association, the National League for Nursing, and Sigma Theta Tau.

Springhouse Corporation
Springhouse, Pennsylvania

Staff

Executive Director, Editorial
Stanley Loeb

Executive Director, Creative Services
Jean Robinson

Director of Trade and Textbooks
Minnie B. Rose, RN, BSN, MEd

Art Director
John Hubbard

Consultant
Maryann Foley, RN, BSN

Acquisitions Editor
Donna L. Hilton, RN, BSN, CEN

Editors
Kevin Law (manager), Judd Howard

Copy Editors
Keith de Pinho, Doris Weinstock

Designers
Stephanie Peters (associate art director),
Jackie Bove Facciolo

Art Production
Robert Perry (manager), Heather Bernhardt,
Anna Brindisi, Donald Knauss, Robert Wieder

Typography
David Kosten (manager), Diane Paluba (assistant
manager), Joyce Rossi Biletz, Elizabeth Bergman,
Robin Rantz, Valerie L. Rosenberger

Manufacturing
Deborah Meiris (manager), T.A. Landis,
Jennifer Suter

Production Coordination
Aline S. Miller (manager), Laurie J. Sander,
Laura L. Williams, Maura Murphy

SN14-011189

Library of Congress Cataloging-in-Publication Data

Innerarity, Sheryl A.
  Fluids and electrolyte management / Sheryl A. Innerarity, June L. Stark.
    p. cm. — (Springhouse notes)
  Includes bibliographical references.
  1. Water—electrolyte imbalances. 2. Water—electrolyte balance (Physiology) 3. Nursing.
    I. Stark, June L. II. Title. III. Series.
    [DNLM: 1. Acid-Base Equilibrium—nurses' instruction. 2. Acid-Base Equilibrium—outlines. 3. Acid-Base Imbalance—nurses' instruction. 4. Acid-Base Imbalance—outlines. 5. Water-Electrolyte Balance—nurses' instruction. 6. Water-Electrolyte Balance—outlines. 7. Water-Electrolyte Imbalance—nurses' instruction. 8 Water-Electrolyte Imbalance—outlines. Qu 18I58F]RC630.I59   1990
616.3'9—dc20
DNLM/DLC
for Library of Congress   89-21583
ISBN 0-87434-228-7   CIP

Contents

How to Use Springhouse Notes

Today, more than ever, nursing students face enormous time pressures. Nursing education has become more sophisticated, increasing the difficulties students have with studying efficiently and keeping pace.

The need for a comprehensive, well-designed series of study aids is great, which is why we've produced Springhouse Notes...to meet that need. Springhouse Notes provide essential course material in outline form, enabling the nursing student to study more effectively, improve understanding, achieve higher test scores, and get better grades.

Key features appear throughout each book, making the information more accessible and easier to remember.
- **Learning Objectives.** These objectives precede each section in the book to help the student evaluate knowledge before and after study.
- **Key Points.** Highlighted in color throughout the book, these points provide a way to quickly review critical information. Key points may include:
—a cardinal sign or symptom of a disorder
—the most current or popular theory about a topic
—a distinguishing characteristic of a disorder
—the most important step of a process
—a critical assessment component
—a crucial nursing intervention
—the most widely used or successful therapy or treatment.
- **Points to Remember.** This information, found at the end of each section, summarizes the section in capsule form.
- **Glossary.** Difficult, frequently used, or sometimes misunderstood terms are defined for the student at the end of each section.

Remember: Springhouse Notes are learning tools designed to *help* you. They are not intended for use as a primary information source. They should never substitute for class attendance, text reading, or classroom note-taking.

This book, *Fluids and Electrolytes,* presents the concepts essential to fluid and electrolyte balance as a framework for discussing water, electrolyte, and acid-base balance and imbalance. Major water, electrolyte, and acid-base imbalances and conditions associated with these imbalances are outlined using a nursing process approach. The section on fluid and electrolyte replacement therapy includes important information on the solutions used in replacement therapy and on specific nursing implications for each type of replacement therapy. Keep in mind that these nursing implications, which generally include more than one option in the progression of care, must be prioritized and adapted to meet individual patient's needs.

Essential Concepts of Fluid and Electrolyte Balance

Learning Objectives

After studying this section, the reader should be able to:

- Describe the characteristics of the homeostatic state.

- Identify the fluid, electrolyte, and pH components found in the intracellular and extracellular compartments.

- Describe how fluids and electrolytes move between the vascular and interstitial spaces.

- State the normal ranges for pH.

I. Essential Concepts of Fluid and Electrolyte Balance

A. Introduction

1. Knowledge of the basic concepts of fluid and electrolyte balance is necessary to provide safe, quality nursing care
2. Fluid and electrolyte balance involves composition and movement of body fluids
3. Body fluids are solutions composed of water and solutes
4. Solutions—liquids (solvents) containing dissolved substances (solutes)—are classified according to their concentration, or *tonicity,* and include:
   a. Isotonic solutions
   b. Hypotonic solutions
   c. Hypertonic solutions
5. Body fluids are isotonic solutions
6. Many diseases and disorders can affect fluid and electrolyte balance
7. Solutions ingested into the body through food, drink, or I.V. fluids also can affect fluid and electrolyte balance

B. Homeostasis

1. General information
   a. Homeostasis refers to the state of internal equilibrium within the body when all body systems are in balance
   b. Homeostasis occurs when fluid, electrolyte, and acid-base balance are all maintained within narrow limits despite a wide variation in dietary intake and metabolic rate
   c. Homeostasis often is referred to as a steady state or as equilibrium
2. Key concepts
   a. Water and solutes are distributed throughout the body's compartments
   b. To maintain homeostasis, water and solutes are in constant movement and are exchanged continuously
   c. When water and solute concentrations are altered within the body, imbalances develop, disrupting homeostasis

C. Water

1. General information
   a. Body fluid is composed primarily of water
   b. Water is the solvent in which all solutes in the body are either dissolved or suspended
   c. An average-sized man (weight 155 lb [70 kg]) has about 40 liters of body water, representing 50% to 60% of total body weight
   d. In women, body water accounts for 45% to 50% of total body weight
   e. Women have lower percentages of total body weight as body water than men because they have a higher percentage of body fat, which does not retain water well
   f. In infants, body water represents about 80% of the total body weight

g. In children, the percentage of total weight as body water decreases steadily until it reaches adult percentages by about age 8
h. Obese persons have lower percentages of total weight as body water because adipose tissue does not retain water well
2. Key concepts
   a. Body water is contained in two major body compartments, the intracellular fluid (ICF) and the extracellular fluid (ECF)
   b. Fluid balance is maintained when water intake equals water output
   c. Normally, fluid balance occurs despite wide variations in daily fluid intake
   d. The primary source of body fluid intake is water ingestion
   e. Water is ingested primarily by drinking fluids and eating foods
   f. All foods contain water; almost 100% of the weight of fruit and vegetables and 70% of the weight of meat is in water
   g. Approximately 350 ml of water is generated daily from digestion and metabolism of carbohydrates, protein, and fat; this is considered intake
   h. Under certain circumstances, water can be introduced to the body parenterally (other than through the GI tract)—usually intravenously

D. Solutes
1. General information
   a. Solutes are substances dissolved in a solution
   b. Solutes are classified as electrolytes or nonelectrolytes
   c. *Nonelectrolytes* are solutes without an electrical charge
   d. Nonelectrolytes found in body fluids include glucose, proteins, oxygen, carbon dioxide, and organic acids
   e. *Electrolytes* are solutes that generate an electrical charge when dissolved in water
   f. Positively charged electrolytes are called *cations*
   g. Major cations in body fluid include sodium (Na), potassium (K), and hydrogen (H)
   h. Negatively charged electrolytes are called *anions*
   i. Major anions in body fluid include chloride (Cl) and bicarbonate (HCO_3)
2. Key concepts
   a. The concentration of various solutes in body fluid varies, depending on the body fluid compartment
   b. Sodium is the major cation in the ECF; potassium is the major cation in the ICF
   c. Electrolytes combine in solutions based on the electrical charge they produce
   d. The chemical combining power of electrolytes is measured in milliequivalents (mEq); 1 mEq of anion reacts chemically with 1 mEq of cation
   e. The total number of cation milliequivalents in body fluids must always equal the total number of anion milliequivalents

    f. Measurement of solute concentration in body fluid is based on the fluid's *osmotic pressure,* expressed as either osmolality or osmolarity

    g. *Osmolality* refers to the number of osmols (the standard unit of osmotic pressure) per kilogram of solution, expressed as milliosmols per kilogram (mOsm/kg)

    h. *Osmolarity* refers to the number of osmols per liter of solution, expressed as mOsm/liter

    i. *Osmolarity* and *osmolality* are commonly used interchangeably; most calculations of body fluid solute concentrations are based on osmolarity

E. Body fluid compartments

  1. General information

    a. Body fluid is divided by semipermeable membranes into two major body compartments, the ICF and ECF

    b. The ICF, representing fluid inside the cells, is the largest body compartment

    c. The ICF accounts for about two-thirds of total body fluid

    d. The ECF accounts for about one-third of total body fluid

    e. The ECF is divided into three separate body compartments: interstitial fluid (ISF), intravascular fluid (plasma), and transcellular water (TSW)

    f. ISF occupies the spaces between the cells; it constitutes 15% of total body fluid

    g. Plasma is found in the intravascular space and constitutes about 4% of total body fluid, or about 75 ml/kg of body weight

    h. TSW constitutes only 1% to 2% of total body fluid and as such sometimes is not considered a separate compartment

    i. TSW is usually found in specialized compartments, such as peritoneal fluid, ocular fluid, cerebrospinal fluid, and synovial fluid

  2. Key concepts

    a. Body fluid is not confined to one defined area or compartment; normal body membranes are permeable to water, which facilitates fluid movement through them

    b. Certain solutes are more abundant in certain body compartments and tend to be limited to this compartment under normal conditions. For example, K is more abundant in the ICF, and Na is more abundant in the ECF

    c. Solute movement from one body fluid compartment to another occurs through various mechanisms, such as active and passive transport

    d. Proteins are solutes usually confined to the plasma that create colloid osmotic pressure in the ECF, affecting fluid and solute movement between the ECF and the ICF

F. Body fluid movement

  1. General information

    a. Constant movement of water and solutes between body fluid compartments maintains homeostasis

    b. Membrane permeability and hydrostatic and osmotic pressures affect water and solute movement

    c. Movement of water and solutes takes place through active and passive transport mechanisms

    d. *Active transport mechanisms* involve chemical activity and the release of energy

    e. *Passive transport mechanisms* do not involve chemical activity or use of energy

    f. Passive transport mechanisms include osmosis and diffusion

2. Key concepts: water movement

    a. All body water movement occurs through *osmosis*

    b. By osmosis a solvent moves through a semipermeable membrane from an area of lower solute concentration to one of higher concentration

    c. Water movement and distribution depend on the concentration of solute (primarily Na) within a compartment—the compartment's osmolality

    d. Water responds to changes in osmolality because it moves freely between compartments under osmotic or hydrostatic pressure

3. Key concepts: solute movement

    a. Solute movement occurs through active and passive transport mechanisms

    b. Solute distribution depends on the concentrations of body fluid compartments

    c. Passive transport of solutes is affected by the electrical potential across cell membranes

    d. By *diffusion* solutes move from an area of higher solute concentration to one of lower concentration, resulting in an equal distribution of solute

    e. *Filtration* requires the force of hydrostatic pressure to move solutes through cell membranes via diffusion; the fluid produced by this process is known as *ultrafiltrate*

    f. Active transport uses an energy source to move solutes from an area of lower solute concentration to one of higher solute concentration against concentration gradient

4. Key concepts: cellular movement of water and solutes

    a. Most solutes move by passive transport mechanisms

    b. Active transport, specifically the *sodium-potassium pump*, is necessary move sodium from the cells to the ECF

    c. The same pump mechanism drives potassium from the ECF into the ce this allows solutes to move from an area of lower solute concentration one of higher solute concentration

    d. Water moves by osmosis from the ECF to the ICF based on the osmolality of the fluid compartment

    e. If the ICF osmolality increases, water will shift from the ECF into the ICF

    f. If the ECF osmolality increases, water will shift from the ICF into the ECF

5. Key concepts: vascular movement of water and solutes

    a. Movement of water and solutes occurs continuously between the vascu and ISF compartments

    b. Movement of water depends on hydrostatic and colloid osmotic pressures in the capillaries; solutes move by diffusion

    c. Pressure differences in the venous and arterial ends of capillaries influence the direction and rate of water and solute movement; this is known as *Starling's law*

    d. Colloid osmotic pressures help maintain plasma volume

    e. Hydrostatic pressure in the arterial end of the capillary is normally +25 mm Hg, favoring movement of plasma water into the ISF

    f. Perivascular tissues exert a pressure of +11 mm Hg, favoring movement of water into the ISF

    g. Both forces together exert a pressure of +36 mm Hg, which is opposed by the combined colloidal osmotic pressure of plasma proteins and albumins, a negative pressure of −28 mm Hg

    h. The remaining net pressure of +8 mm Hg encourages the movement of water, solutes, and gases from the vascular space to the ISF

    i. Hydrostatic pressure in the venous end of the capillary is normally +10 mm Hg (because the venous end is farther from the heart than the arterial end)

    j. Interstitial pressure remains +11 mm Hg; the combination of positive venous pressures equals 21 mm Hg, favoring movement of water out of the capillary

    k. Plasma proteins exert an opposing pressure of −28 mm Hg, resulting in a total net negative pressure of −7 mm Hg

    l. The negative force draws water, metabolic cellular wastes, and carbon dioxide from the ISF into the vascular compartment, resulting in eventual degradation and removal of these substances by a major organ system, such as the lungs or kidneys

G. Body fluid pH

  1. General information

    a. The term *pH* refers to the acidity or alkalinity of a solution, which is determined by the hydrogen ion concentration

    b. Hydrogen ion donors are considered *acids*

    c. Hydrogen ion acceptors are considered *bases*

    d. pH regulation is affected by the dilution of products of metabolism by large volumes of body fluids

    e. All body fluids have a pH; the normal pH of different body fluids varies

    f. The body fluid pH commonly measured to determine acid-base balance is arterial blood pH

    g. Arterial blood pH is regulated through the action of buffers, the lungs, (via K ion exchange), and the kidneys, in that order

  2. Key concepts

    a. Normal arterial blood pH ranges between 7.35 to 7.45

    b. Despite continuous additions of metabolites from cells and food, arterial blood pH usually is maintained at a fairly constant level

    c. An arterial blood pH of ≤6.8 or ≥7.8 is incompatible with life

Points to Remember

Homeostasis exists when the intake of fluid and electrolytes equals the output.

Extreme gains or losses of fluids, electrolytes, or acid-base components result in an imbalanced state.

The intracellular fluid (ICF) compartment is composed of fluid within cells; the extracellular fluid compartment (ECF) is composed of the interstitial, intravascular, and transcellular spaces.

Body water and solutes move continuously between the ICF and the ECF.

Body water moves by osmosis; solutes move via passive or active transport mechanisms.

Body fluid pH reflects hydrogen ion concentration.

Glossary

Body fluid—fluid composed of water and solutes and contained in the ICF and ECF compartments

Buffer—substance that minimizes pH changes by absorbing hydrogen ions when a base is added to the system and releasing hydrogen ions when an acid is added

Electrolyte—element or compound that, when melted or dissolved in water or another solvent, dissociates into ions that carry an electrical charge

Hydrostatic pressure—pressure exerted by a liquid

Osmolality—osmotic pressure of a solution expressed in milliosmols per kilogram of solution

Osmolarity—the osmotic pressure of a solution expressed in milliosmols per liter of solution

Transcellular water—highly specialized fluid found in specific areas, such as gastric juices and cerebrospinal fluid

Water Balance

Learning Objectives

After studying this section, the reader should be able to:

- State the normal range of serum osmolality.

- Describe the relationship between sodium and water balance.

- Discuss the process of body water regulation.

- Describe the difference between sensible and insensible water losses.

- List nursing implications for assessing fluid status.

II. Water Balance

A. Introduction

1. Water, the most abundant component of body fluid, is required in adequate amounts for body function
2. Water is used by the body to:
   a. Act as a solvent for many body chemicals
   b. Aid various chemical reactions
   c. Maintain stability of body fluids
   d. Aid nutrient transport to cells
   e. Provide a medium for waste excretion
   f. Act as a lubricant between cells to permit friction-free movement
   g. Aid body temperature regulation through perspiration
3. The body gains and loses water each day; gains and losses must be balanced to maintain body fluid balance
4. Monitoring fluid intake and output is a valuable tool for determining homeostasis
5. Nursing implications for water balance
   a. Carefully monitor fluid intake and output
   b. When monitoring output, calculate sensible (measurable) losses and estimate insensible losses as closely as possible
   c. In patients for whom measuring urine output is difficult or impossible, estimate output through other means, such as weighing urine-soaked diapers or incontinence pads, then subtracting the weight of a dry diaper or pad, and converting the weight of urine to a volume measurement
   d. For a patient with watery diarrhea, estimate fluid loss by using a bedside commode, bedpan, or other collection device
   e. Obtain hourly output measurements, if necessary, to identify a pattern of urine output
   f. Monitor for anuria, oliguria, or polyuria, which may signal serious problems requiring medical intervention
   g. Remember, daily weight is an accurate measure of fluid balance; a history of a patient's weight gain or loss can be used to assess fluid, sodium, and caloric intake
   h. To ensure accuracy, obtain daily weights using the same scale, before breakfast, and when the patient has an empty bladder
   i. Correlate daily weight with the 24-hour intake and output, with +500 ml equaling a 1-lb weight gain and −500 ml equaling a 1-lb weight loss
   j. Document use of all medications, both over-the-counter and prescription, to anticipate potential fluid-related complications
   k. Monitor urine specific gravity and color: a specific gravity ≤1.010 and light-colored, dilute urine may indicate overhydration; a specific gravity ≥1.030 and dark-colored, concentrated urine may point to dehydration

l. Remember, a falsely elevated or depressed specific gravity may occur after administration of radiopaque dyes or diuretics, respectively

m. Be aware that specific gravity is not reliable if the patient has renal disease associated with a concentration defect

n. Monitor specific diagnostic tests, such as serum and urine osmolality, blood urea nitrogen, hematocrit, and creatinine, to evaluate water balance

B. Water intake

1. General information

a. Water must be supplied regularly for metabolic use and to compensate for fluid losses

b. The total daily intake of water is approximately 2,500 ml

c. The primary source of water is ingested liquids, which account for approximately 1,500 ml/day

d. Water also is obtained by ingesting solid foods, which account for approximately 800 ml/day

e. Food oxidation provides an additional source of water intake, accounting for approximately 300 ml/day

f. If water cannot be ingested orally, it may be given intravenously in fluids that closely resemble the composition of body fluids

---

DAILY FLUID GAINS AND LOSSES

In a healthy person, the fluids ingested balance the fluids excreted (see illustration below). Water loss via the skin and lungs will increase in a hot, dry environment or with increased respiratory rate, fever, or skin injury (such as burns). Water loss via the kidneys varies largely with the amount of solute excreted and with the level of antidiuretic hormone, which controls the kidneys' reabsorption of water.

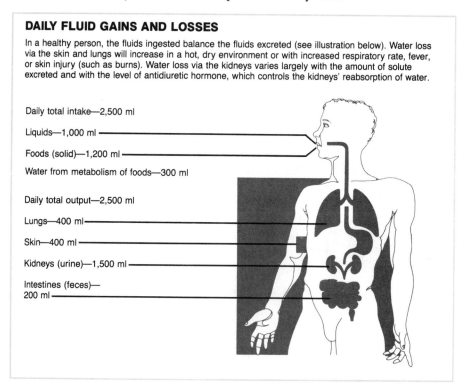

Daily total intake—2,500 ml

Liquids—1,000 ml

Foods (solid)—1,200 ml

Water from metabolism of foods—300 ml

Daily total output—2,500 ml

Lungs—400 ml

Skin—400 ml

Kidneys (urine)—1,500 ml

Intestines (feces)—200 ml

2. Control mechanisms
    a. Water intake is regulated primarily by the thirst sensation
    b. Thirst is stimulated by local responses, such as dry mouth, and systemic responses, such as the action of antidiuretic hormone
    c. Water intake also depends on access to water and the ability to drink it

C. Water regulation

1. General information
    a. Water regulation helps maintain a serum osmolality of 280 to 295 mOsm/liter
    b. Water regulation is always associated with sodium regulation
    c. Regulation of water balance is accomplished by the kidneys, the adrenal cortex, the thirst mechanism, and the secretion or inhibition of antidiuretic hormone (ADH) (see "Sodium [Na]" in Section III for more information)
2. Control mechanisms
    a. Thirst alerts the body to a fluid deficit
    b. The center for thirst control is located in the anterior hypothalamus
    c. Osmoreceptor cells in the hypothalamus sense changes in serum osmolality and initiate impulses to produce the thirst sensation and the release of ADH
    d. Hormonal control of extracellular osmolality is provided by the release or inhibition of ADH, which is produced by the hypothalamus and stored in the posterior pituitary gland
    e. Normal serum osmolality inhibits ADH release, which allows water excretion in the renal tubules
    f. Increased serum osmolality stimulates ADH release, which promotes water reabsorption by the kidneys

D. Water conservation

1. General information
    a. The body can conserve water when intake does not equal output
    b. The mechanisms that regulate water balance also can conserve water under adverse conditions
2. Control mechanisms
    a. Intracellular dehydration stimulates the osmoreceptor cells of the hypothalamus to initiate the thirst sensation
    b. Extracellular dehydration, increased serum osmolality, or a decrease in circulating blood volume also stimulates the hypothalamus to initiate the thirst sensation

    c. An increase in serum osmolality of 1% to 2% (which indicates a water deficit) causes increased secretion of ADH from the posterior pituitary gland to promote water reabsorption in the renal tubules

    d. A decrease in circulating blood volume stimulates the cardiac atrial receptors, which in turn promote ADH release, resulting in increased water reabsorption by the kidneys and increased circulating blood volume

    e. Angiotensin II, an end product of renin activation, stimulates secretion of aldosterone from the adrenal cortex

    f. Aldosterone secretion is regulated by a decrease in circulating blood volume and results in sodium reabsorption by the kidneys

    g. Because sodium and water are closely related, this sodium reabsorption also results in water reabsorption

E. Water excretion

  1. General information

    a. Water is excreted from the body through the kidneys, skin, lungs, and GI tract

    b. Water losses can be categorized as sensible or insensible losses

    c. Sensible losses are through urine; insensible losses include water lost through the skin, respiratory system, and GI tract

    d. Sensible or insensible losses affect the extracellular fluid immediately and, if not replaced, will eventually affect the intracellular fluid

  2. Control mechanisms

    a. The kidneys are the major regulatory organs of water balance

    b. Adults lose between 1 and 2 liters of water as urine each day; the amount of urine produced by the kidneys is influenced by ADH and aldosterone levels

    c. Urine excretion should equal about 1 ml per kilogram of body weight per hour in any age-group

    d. The kidneys have the ability to produce urine with a wide range in osmolality; the range of normal specific gravity is 1.003 to 1.030.

    e. The kidneys can excrete urine with a range in osmolality of 200 to 1,400 mOsm/liter without a change in the amount of metabolic wastes or solutes filtered by the tubules

    f. Water loss through perspiration can approach 600 ml/day

    g. The lungs may eliminate 300 to 400 ml of water daily through respiration; increased respiratory rate and depth cause increased water losses

    h. About 200 ml of water are excreted in feces daily; such water losses may be much greater during GI illness

Points to Remember

Water is the main component of body fluid.

Water balance and sodium balance are closely related.

Water balance and sodium balance are regulated by the kidneys, the adrenal cortex, antidiuretic hormone (ADH), aldosterone, and the thirst mechanism.

Monitoring body weight is the most accurate method of assessing fluid status.

The volume and concentration of the urine usually reflect the body's water balance.

Intake and output records provide an estimate of the 24-hour fluid balance.

Glossary

Anuria—daily urine output of less than 50 ml

Extracellular dehydration—water deficit in the extracellular compartment

Intracellular dehydration—water deficit in the intracellular compartment

Oliguria—daily urine output between 50 to 400 ml

Osmoreceptor cells—specialized cells in the hypothalamus that respond to serum osmolality and trigger the thirst sensation

Polyuria—urine output greater than fluid intake

Specific gravity—weight of a substance in relation to the weight of an equal volume of water. Normal urine specific gravity ranges from 1.003 to 1.030; water is considered to have a specific gravity of 1.000

Electrolyte Balance

Learning Objectives

After studying this section, the reader should be able to:

• Describe the characteristics of an electrolyte.

• List the major intracellular and extracellular electrolytes.

• State the functions of sodium, potassium, and calcium.

• List the electrolytes that play a role in normal cardiac function.

III. Electrolyte Balance

A. Introduction

1. Electrolytes, electrically charged solutes in body fluids, are necessary to maintain life
2. Electrolytes perform four essential functions
   a. Promote neuromuscular irritability
   b. Maintain body fluid osmolality
   c. Regulate acid-base balance
   d. Regulate distribution of body fluids among body fluid compartments
3. Electrolyte imbalance—abnormal excess or deficit of an electrolyte in body fluids—can cause illness
4. Nurses must be aware of the normal functions and levels of electrolytes in the body to better assess and monitor fluid and electrolyte balance in patients
5. Nursing implications for assessing electrolyte balance
   a. Assess overall fluid balance by monitoring daily weight, fluid intake and output, and urine specific gravity; fluid balance is closely related to electrolyte balance (See Appendix A: *Fluid Balance Checklist,* pages 108-110)
   b. Assess neurologic status, specifically for altered level of consciousness, which may result from an electrolyte imbalance
   c. Evaluate motor and sensory function, especially deep tendon reflexes; neuromuscular irritability may indicate electrolyte imbalances
   d. Monitor vital signs, especially pulse and blood pressure; certain electrolytes—such as sodium (Na), potassium (K), and magnesium (Mg)—directly affect pulse and blood pressure regulation
   e. Compare ongoing ECG readings with the patient's baseline ECG to detect changes that may indicate an imbalance
   f. Assess respiratory status for changes in rate, depth, and character
   g. Monitor serum electrolyte levels for abnormalities
   h. Remember, electrolytes may be obtained through food intake; be aware of fluids and foods high in certain electrolytes
   i. Assess nutritional status by monitoring dietary intake and weight; obtain anthropometric measurements and compare to standards
   j. Evaluate the patient's health history for medical conditions that might alter electrolyte balance
   k. Evaluate the patient's medication history for prescription and over-the-counter drugs that could interfere with electrolyte balance, such as diuretics, antacids, and salt substitutes

B. Sodium (Na)

1. General information
   a. Na is the major cation in the extracellular fluid (ECF)
   b. Normal serum Na concentration in the ECF ranges from 136 to 145 mEq/liter

NORMAL ELECTROLYTE CONCENTRATION LEVELS IN INTRACELLULAR AND EXTRACELLULAR FLUID

Blood contains both intracellular fluid (blood in red blood cells) and extracellular fluid (plasma fluid). Because their cells allow different substances to permeate, intracellular and extracellular fluids have different electrolyte concentration levels. Be aware that standards for these values vary among institutions.
Note: In the clinical setting, the nurse will see values reflecting the components of extracellular fluid only.

ELECTROLYTE	INTRACELLULAR CONCENTRATION	EXTRACELLULAR CONCENTRATION
Sodium	10 mEq/liter	136 to 146 m Eq/liter
Potassium	140 mEq/liter	3.5 to 5.5 mEq/liter
Calcium	10 mEq/liter	4.5 to 5.8 mEq/liter
Magnesium	40 mEq/liter	1.6 to 2.2 mEq/liter
Chloride	4 mEq/liter	96 to 106 mEq/liter
Phosphate	100 mEq/liter	1 to 1.5 mEq/liter

    c. Normal Na concentration in the intracellular fluid (ICF) is 10 mEq/liter
    d. Excretion or absorption of Na usually involves proportionate excretion or absorption of water and chloride (Cl)
    e. Although the minimum daily Na requirement is 2 g, adults in the United States consume an average of 6 g/day
  2. Functions
    a. Maintains appropriate ECF osmolality
    b. Maintains ECF volume and influences body water distribution (with Cl)
    c. Affects the concentration, excretion, and absorption of K and Cl
    d. Combines readily with bicarbonate (HCO_3) and Cl to help regulate acid-base balance
    e. Aids impulse transmission in nerve and muscle fibers
  3. Regulation
    a. Na balance is regulated mainly by the kidneys, primarily through aldosterone action
    b. The kidneys can adjust Na excretion to match Na intake despite great variations in Na intake
    c. The Na level in the ECF is controlled by a feedback loop, in which aldosterone secretion by the adrenal cortex stimulates the renal tubules to reabsorb Na
    d. A change in serum Na level usually reflects a change in total body water balance
    e. Increased Na level in the ECF results in decreased aldosterone production, which increases renal Na excretion

     f. Increased Na level in the ECF also raises ECF osmolality, which stimulates antidiuretic hormone (ADH) release that increases renal water reabsorption

     g. Decreased Na level in the ECF results in increased aldosterone production, which decreases renal Na excretion

     h. Decreased Na level in the ECF also lowers ECF osmolality, which inhibits ADH release and increases renal water excretion

C. Potassium (K)

1. General information
   a. K is the major cation in the ICF
   b. Normal serum K level ranges from 3.5 to 5.5 mEq/liter
   c. Cellular K concentration (usually not measured clinically) is 140 to 145 mEq/liter
   d. The daily dietary requirement of K is about 40 mEq; the average daily intake is 60 to 100 mEq

2. Functions
   a. Maintains cell electroneutrality and cell osmolality
   b. Directly affects cardiac muscle contraction and electrical conductivity
   c. Aids neuromuscular transmission of nerve impulses
   d. Plays a major role in acid-base balance; any alteration in K balance will result in acid-base imbalance

3. Regulation
   a. K must be ingested daily because the body does not conserve it
   b. The kidneys eliminate about 80% of ingested K; about 20 to 40 mEq is lost in each liter of urine
   c. Remaining K is excreted in feces; 5 to 10 mEq is lost in each liter of GI fluid
   d. K and Na have a reciprocal relationship; the feedback mechanism regulating Na excretion is opposite that regulating K excretion
   e. Aldosterone secretion results in renal Na reabsorption and renal K excretion
   f. Because K ions are exchanged for hydrogen (H) ions in acid-base balances, a decrease in K excretion accompanies an increase in H ion excretion; the opposite is also true
   g. The serum K level rises in acidosis and falls in alkalosis; thus, fluctuating serum K levels may or may not reflect an absolute increase or decrease in the total body K level

D. Chloride (Cl)

1. General information
   a. Cl is the major anion in the ECF
   b. Normal serum Cl level ranges from 96 to 106 mEq/liter

2. Functions
   a. Maintains serum osmolality (along with Na)

      b. Combines with major cations to create important compounds, such as sodium chloride (NaCl), hydrochloric acid (HCl), potassium chloride (KCl), and calcium chloride (CaCl)

      c. Through production of HCl, Cl plays a major role in maintaining acid-base balance

  3. Regulation

      a. Cl balance is tied most closely to Na balance

      b. Cl and Na levels usually change in direct proportion to one another

      c. Decreased Cl level (most commonly due to GI losses) results in increased HCO_3 level to balance anions and cations in the ECF

E. Calcium (Ca)

  1. General information

      a. Ca is the major cation involved in the structure and function of teeth and bones

      b. About 50% of serum Ca exists in the ionized form and is chemically active; this amount is measured as serum Ca

      c. The remaining serum Ca is bound to serum proteins, particularly albumin; because any change in serum protein levels affects the total serum Ca level, the albumin level must be considered with the Ca level

      d. Ca and phosphorus (P) have an inverse relationship; increased serum Ca level results in decreased serum P level, and decreased serum Ca level results in increased serum P level

      e. The recommended daily dietary Ca intake is 800 mg

      f. Normal serum Ca level ranges from 8.5 to 10.5 mEq/dl (4 to 5.5 mEq/liter)

      g. Normal Ca concentration in the ICF is 10 mEq/liter

  2. Functions

      a. Enhances bone strength and durability (along with P)

      b. Helps maintain cell membrane structure, function, and membrane permeability

      c. Affects activation, excitation, and contraction of cardiac and skeletal muscle

      d. Participates in neurotransmitter release at synapses

      e. Helps activate specific steps in blood coagulation

      f. Activates serum complement, a major factor in immune system function

  3. Regulation

      a. Ca is absorbed in the small intestine in the presence of vitamin D

      b. Vitamin D promotes Ca absorption; P inhibits Ca absorption

      c. Ca absorption occurs because of 1,25-dihydroxycholecalciferol (calcitriol); 1,25 DCH is activated vitamin D

      d. Parathyroid hormone (PTH) promotes Ca transfer from bone to plasma and aids intestinal and renal Ca absorption

      e. Decreased Ca level in the ECF directly stimulates PTH release from the parathyroid glands, which releases calcium phosphate ($CaPO_4$) from bone and indirectly activates mechanisms to increase Ca reabsorption and P excretion from the renal tubules and the GI tract

f. Ca transfer from plasma to bone is aided by calcitonin, which directly lowers serum Ca levels

g. Elevated Ca level in the ECF stimulates the thyroid gland to release calcitonin, which inhibits Ca release from bone and reduces PTH production and release, thereby decreasing mobilization, intestinal absorption, and Ca reabsorption by the kidneys

h. Almost 50% of serum Ca is bound to serum albumin; thus, albumin levels must be considered with Ca levels

i. When serum becomes alkaline, more Ca binds to protein; thus, symptoms of hypocalcemia usually occur during alkalosis

j. Renal excretion of Ca is limited by calcitriol in deficiency states

F. Phosphorus (P)
1. General information
    a. P is a major anion in the ICF
    b. About 80% of P exists in bone in combination with Ca (in a 1:2 ratio of P to C)
    c. Normal serum P level ranges from 2.5 to 4.5 mEq/dl (1 to 1.5 mEq/liter)
    d. Normal P concentration in the ICF is 100 mEq/liter
2. Functions
    a. Is an essential component of bones and teeth (with Ca)
    b. Helps maintain cell membrane integrity
    c. Plays a major role in acid-base balance through its action as a urinary buffer (600 to 900 mg is excreted in the urine daily)
    d. Plays essential roles in muscle, red blood cell, and neurologic function and in carbohydrate, protein, and fat metabolism
    e. Functions in cellular metabolism to promote energy transfer to cells
3. Regulation
    a. PTH affects P level by influencing renal excretion of P and increasing Ca reabsorption in response to decreased Ca level in the ECF
    b. Mobilization of P from bone is influenced by PTH levels (see Section III.E.3 for more information)

G. Magnesium (Mg)
1. General information
    a. Mg is a major cation in the ICF, closely related to Ca and P
    b. About 60% of Mg is contained in bone
    c. A normal diet supplies approximately 25 mEq of Mg daily; of this amount, 10 mEq is absorbed through the small bowel, 10 mEq is excreted in urine, and the remainder is excreted in feces
    d. Normal serum Mg level ranges from 1.5 to 2.5 mEq/liter, with 33% bound to protein and the remainder existing as free cations
    e. Normal Mg concentration in the ICF is 40 mEq/liter
2. Functions
    a. Activates intracellular enzymes and acts in carbohydrate and protein metabolism

  b. Acts on the myoneural junction, affecting neuromuscular irritability and contractility of cardiac and skeletal muscle
  c. Affects peripheral vasodilation, resulting in changes in blood pressure and cardiac output
  d. Facilitates transport of Na and K across cell membranes
  e. Influences intracellular Ca level through its effect on PTH secretion
3. Regulation
  a. Control of Mg is not clearly understood
  b. Factors that influence Ca and K balance seem to act on Mg as well
  c. Signs and symptoms of Mg imbalance—particularly hypomagnesemia—mimic those of Ca imbalance, which may interfere with diagnosis and treatment of Mg imbalance
  d. The kidneys can conserve Mg efficiently, restricting losses to 1 mEq/day if necessary; however, excessive Mg excretion can result from diuretic use

Points to Remember

Sodium (Na) is the major cation in the ECF.

Potassium (K) is the major cation in the ICF.

Renal and hormonal systems are the major regulators of all electrolytes.

Normal ranges of serum electrolyte levels are as follows: Na, 136 to 145 mEq/liter; K, 3.5 to 5 mEq/liter; Cl, 96 to 106 mEq/liter; Ca, 8.5 to 10.5 mEq/dl; P, 2.5 to 4.5 mEq/dl; Mg, 1.5 to 2.5 mEq/liter.

Glossary

Aldosterone—adrenocortical hormone that regulates Na and K balance

Buffer—substance that absorbs or releases H ions in response to an acid-base imbalance

Ion—solute with a positive or negative electrical charge; positively charged ions are known as cations, and negatively charged ions are known as anions

Myoneural junction—area of contact between the ends of a large myelinated nerve fiber and a skeletal muscle fiber

Acid-Base Balance

Learning Objectives

After studying this section, the reader should be able to:

• Describe the characteristics of an acid and a base.

• State the alterations in pH that occur in acidosis and in alkalosis.

• Describe the roles of the renal and respiratory systems in buffering and regulating acid-base balance.

• Identify the normal values for an arterial blood gas analysis.

• Describe renal and respiratory compensation.

IV. Acid-Base Balance

A. Introduction

1. Acid-base balance refers to homeostasis of the hydrogen (H) ion concentration in body fluids

2. Body fluids are classified as acids or bases according to their H ion concentration
   a. An acid is an H ion donor
   b. A base is an H ion acceptor

3. Acid-base balance is maintained by controlling the H ion concentration of body fluids, specifically extracellular fluid (ECF)
   a. The concentration of H ions in a body fluid is expressed as the pH
   b. The numerical value of the pH is inversely proportional to the number of H ions in solution; the pH falls as the H ion concentration rises. The reverse is also true.

4. Normal blood pH ranges from 7.35 to 7.45; a pH below 6.8 or above 7.8 is incompatible with life

5. *Acidosis* defines an excess of H ions as either acid excess or base deficit and is marked by pH <7.35

6. *Alkalosis* defines a deficit of H ions as either base excess or acid deficit and is marked by pH >7.45

7. A patient's acid-base balance is evaluated by blood gas analysis of either arterial or capillary (in children) blood

B. Measurement of acid-base balance

1. General information
   a. Because acids and bases leave the body mainly through gas exchange between the cells and the external environment, measurement of these gases reflects acid-base balance
   b. Blood gas measurements are the major diagnostic tool for evaluating acid-base balance
   c. Commonly used blood gas measurements include arterial blood gas (ABG) and mixed venous blood gas measurements
   d. Related methods of measurement include transcutaneous blood gas measurements, pulse oximetry, serum anion gap measurements, serum potassium (K) levels, and total carbon dioxide (CO_2) and chloride (Cl) levels
   e. ABG levels are analyzed in blood samples obtained from an artery, such as the radial, brachial, or femoral artery, or from an arterial line; mixed venous blood gas levels are analyzed in blood samples taken from a pulmonary artery catheter or a central venous catheter

2. ABG measurements
   a. ABG levels help determine a patient's acid-base status, evaluate pulmonary gas exchange efficiency, assess the respiratory system, evaluate blood oxygenation, and monitor respiratory therapy

b. ABG measurements include six parameters: pH, partial pressure of CO_2 in arterial blood ($PaCO_2$), bicarbonate (HCO_3) concentration, base excess, partial pressure of oxygen in arterial blood (PaO_2), and oxygen saturation (O_2Sat or SaO_2)

c. pH indicates blood acidity; values >7.45 indicate alkalosis, and values <7.35 indicate acidosis

d. A normal or borderline pH may indicate a normal acid-base balance or the body's attempts at compensating for a slightly abnormal or chronic acid-base imbalance

e. $PaCO_2$ levels indicate the partial pressure of CO_2 in arterial blood and are used to evaluate the respiratory acid-base component

f. $PaCO_2$ values >45 mm Hg indicate hypoventilation or excessive CO_2 retention (hypercapnia) and, therefore, acidosis; values <35 mm Hg indicate hyperventilation or excessive CO_2 exhalation (hypocapnia) and, therefore, alkalosis

g. HCO_3 levels reflect the arterial blood's bicarbonate concentration and are used to evaluate the metabolic acid-base component

h. HCO_3 values >26 mEq/liter indicate alkalosis; values <22 mEq/liter indicate acidosis

i. Base excess reflects the level of HCO_3 and other bases, such as plasma proteins and hemoglobin, and is used to evaluate the metabolic acid-base component

j. Base excess values $>+2$ indicate a base excess (acid deficit) in metabolic alkalosis; values <-2 indicate a base deficit (acid excess) in metabolic acidosis

k. PaO_2 and SaO_2 levels are secondary parameters in assessing acid-base status

l. PaO_2 levels reflect the partial pressure of oxygen in arterial blood, revealing the lungs' ability to oxygenate blood

m. PaO_2 levels are not used to evaluate acid-base status

NORMAL ABG VALUES

The normal values shown below may vary slightly from one laboratory to another, depending on testing methods used. These values apply to adults at sea level.

PARAMETER	NORMAL RANGE
pH	7.35 to 7.45
$PaCO_2$	38 to 45 mm Hg
HCO_3	22 to 26 mEq/liter
Base excess	-2 to $+2$
PaO_2	80 to 100 mm Hg
SaO_2	95% to 100%

   n. PaO$_2$ values <80 mm Hg indicate hypoxemia (for each year over age 60, subtract 1 mm Hg from the normal PaO$_2$ range to determine the normal range for a patient of that age)
   o. SaO$_2$ levels reflect the oxygen-carrying capacity of hemoglobin and help evaluate respiratory function
       (See Appendix C: *Arterial Blood Gas Findings and Interpretations,* page 113)
3. Mixed venous blood gas measurements
   a. Measuring mixed venous blood gases is an increasingly common method of assessing acid-base balance
   b. Mixed venous blood gas measurement reflects the blood gas composition in the alveoli
   c. It also reflects pulmonary capillary ventilation and perfusion
   d. Mixed venous blood gas measurements include six parameters: pH, partial pressure of CO$_2$ in mixed venous blood (P$\bar{v}$CO$_2$), bicarbonate concentration (HCO$_3$), base excess, partial pressure of oxygen in mixed venous blood (P$\bar{v}$O$_2$), and oxygen saturation in mixed venous blood (S$\bar{v}$O$_2$)
   e. Most mixed venous blood gas measurement values are similar to and correlate well with ABGs if the patient's cardiac output remains relatively constant

NORMAL MIXED VENOUS BLOOD GAS VALUES

The normal values shown below may vary slightly from one laboratory to another, depending on testing methods used. These values apply to adults at sea level.

PARAMETER	NORMAL RANGE
pH	7.39 to 7.41
P$\bar{v}$CO$_2$	41 to 51 mm Hg
HCO$_3$	22 to 26 mEq/liter
Base excess	−2 to +2
P$\bar{v}$O$_2$	35 to 40 mm Hg
S$\bar{v}$O$_2$	70% to 75%

C. Buffer regulation of acid-base balance
1. General information
   a. Despite continuous additions of metabolites from cells and food, body pH is maintained at a fairly constant level; H ion concentration is affected by dilution of products of metabolism by large volumes of water
   b. Metabolism produces 50 to 100 ions of H daily and about 15,000 mmol of CO$_2$ daily
   c. The kidneys excrete only 1% of this amount; the lungs and other buffers handle the rest

     d. The cells function as buffers by taking up or releasing extra H ions; this process involves exchanging K for H and thus affects K balance

     e. Buffers regulate H ion concentration by taking up or releasing H or hydroxyl ions

     f. Buffers temporarily minimize the effect of H or HCO_3 on blood pH until the renal or respiratory system takes effect

  2. Carbonic acid and sodium bicarbonate as buffers

     a. The major extracellular chemical buffers are carbonic acid (H_2CO_3) and sodium bicarbonate ($NaHCO_3$)

     b. These buffers are the first to react to a change in pH, but their effect is relatively brief

     c. Bicarbonate acts to maintain a ratio of 20 parts HCO_3 to 1 part H_2CO_3, maintaining blood pH at 7.45

     d. Bicarbonate buffering action is expressed by the equation $CO_2 + H_2O \rightleftharpoons H_2CO_3 \rightleftharpoons H + HCO_3$

     e. The lungs retain or eliminate CO_2, increasing or decreasing H_2CO_3 concentration

  3. Phosphate buffers

     a. Phosphates act as buffers in essentially the same way as the HCO_3-H_2CO_3 system

     b. They play an important role in regulating pH in red blood cells and renal tubular fluids

     c. Monosodium or potassium phosphates are buffers; concentrations are regulated by the kidneys

  4. Protein buffers

     a. Protein buffers are the most abundant buffers in body cells and blood

     b. Oxyhemoglobin gives up its oxygen to the body cells to become reduced hemoglobin, which combines with H ion levels to form a weak acid and thereby act as a buffer

     c. Acid proteinate and neutral proteins also function as buffers

D. Respiratory system regulation and compensation

  1. General information

     a. The lungs are the first line of protection in acid-base regulation, capable of responding to changes within minutes

     b. Alteration in pulmonary function or cessation of respirations usually results in acid-base imbalances

  2. Regulation

     a. The lungs regulate H ion concentration by eliminating CO_2 (which combines with water to form H_2CO_3)

     b. Excessive H_2CO_3 is reduced in the lungs to H_2O and CO_2, which is excreted during breathing

     c. H_2CO_3 in the alveolar capillaries crosses into the alveoli and is broken down into CO_2 and water (H_2O), thereby eliminating an H ion; the reverse reaction also occurs

    d. This is accomplished by adjusting the rate and depth of ventilation in response to the CO_2 level in the blood ($PaCO_2$)

    e. Increased $PaCO_2$ level or low pH results in an increased respiratory rate and *hyperventilation,* causing increased exhalation of CO_2 and thus raising blood pH

    f. Decreased $PaCO_2$ level or high pH results in a decreased respiratory rate and *hypoventilation,* causing CO_2 retention and thus lowering blood pH

  3. Compensation

    a. The lungs can compensate for metabolic disturbances by either retaining or removing CO_2, minimizing the change in serum pH

    b. HCO_3 excess (metabolic alkalosis) suppresses the rate and depth of respirations, causing CO_2 retention and H_2CO_3 buildup

    c. HCO_3 deficit (metabolic acidosis) causes increased rate and depth of respirations and greater elimination of CO_2

E. Renal system regulation and compensation

  1. General information

    a. The renal system is the slowest of all the regulating systems; it takes from a few hours to several days to adjust to changes

    b. The kidneys excrete only 1% of the H ion excess, so they are slow to compensate for acid-base imbalances, usually requiring 24 to 48 hours

    c. The renal system, however, can permanently adjust blood pH

    d. Normal renal regulation involves reactions in the renal tubules: K secretion, Na and HCO_3 reabsorption into the body, and H secretion into the tubules

  2. Regulation

    a. The kidneys may excrete either acidic or alkaline urine to compensate for excesses, but the urine is usually acid

    b. The kidneys reabsorb HCO_3 from the renal tubules in a state of acid excess and excrete HCO_3 in a state of acid deficit

    c. H ions combine with phosphates and are excreted as phosphoric acid to conserve Na and K; H ions are removed and HCO_3 is added to the blood

    d. The kidneys regulate H ion concentration by combining H with ammonia (NH_3) to form ammonium (NH_4); the reverse reaction is also true

    e. In the formation of NH_4, H is removed and HCO_3 is added to the blood

    f. NH_4 is excreted when H ions must be eliminated

  3. Compensation

    a. The kidneys compensate for respiratory imbalances by excreting or retaining H and HCO_3

    b. In H_2CO_3 excess, the kidneys excrete H and conserve HCO_3 to restore balance

    c. In H_2CO_3 deficit, the kidneys retain H and excrete HCO_3 to restore balance

    d. H is exchanged for K to raise or lower the pH

Points to Remember

Normal blood pH ranges from 7.35 to 7.45.

Hydrogen ion content in the body determines pH.

A hydrogen ion excess or a base deficit results in acidosis.

A hydrogen ion deficit or a base excess results in alkalosis.

ABG levels are evaluated to monitor blood pH and to evaluate acid-base imbalances.

Glossary

Acid—substance that is an H ion donor

Acidosis—abnormal state resulting from the gain of H ion donors or H ion acceptors

Alkalosis—abnormal state resulting from the loss of H ion donors or H ion acceptors

Base—substance that is an H ion acceptor

Water Imbalances

Learning Objectives

After studying this section, the reader should be able to:

• Describe the difference between an isotonic water imbalance and an osmotic water imbalance.

• List the clinical manifestations of each type of water imbalance.

• Discuss nursing implications for each type of water imbalance.

• Describe patients at greatest risk for water imbalances.

V. Water Imbalances

A. Introduction

1. Imbalances in body fluids are of two basic types: volume (or isotonic) and osmotic
2. Volume imbalances primarily affect the extracellular fluid (ECF) and involve relatively equal losses or gains of sodium and water
3. Osmotic imbalances primarily affect the intracellular fluid (ICF) and involve relatively unequal losses or gains of sodium and water

B. Extracellular fluid volume deficit (isotonic fluid volume deficit)

1. General information
   a. ECF volume deficit—commonly referred to as *dehydration*—results from relatively equal losses of sodium (Na) and water
   b. Volume losses occur from the ECF, but because the Na to water ratio remains essentially unchanged, osmolality is not affected
   c. Because osmolality is unchanged, regulatory mechanisms—such as antidiuretic hormone (ADH) and aldosterone secretion—are not activated and fluid ordinarily does not shift from the ICF to the ECF
2. Etiology
   a. Prolonged vomiting or gastric suction
   b. Excessive diarrhea
   c. Hemorrhage
   d. Profound urine loss, such as polyuria from diabetic ketoacidosis or diuresis
   e. Fever
   f. Third-space shifting
3. Clinical manifestations
   a. Weight loss
   b. Hypotension
   c. Orthostatic hypotension
   d. Tachycardia
   e. Oliguria
   f. Decreased skin turgor
   g. Dry, furrowed tongue
   h. Soft eyeballs (can be detected by applying gentle pressure on top of the eyelid)
   i. Sticky oral mucosa
   j. Altered level of consciousness (LOC)
   k. Slow-filling jugular veins
4. Diagnostic findings
   a. Increased urine specific gravity
   b. Increased hematocrit
   c. Increased serum protein level
   d. Increased blood urea nitrogen (BUN) level
   e. Normal serum sodium level (usually)

f. Normal serum creatinine level in relation to an elevated BUN level
5. Nursing implications
    a. Monitor fluid intake and output to determine the need for replacement therapy
    b. Check daily weight to note loss that may indicate fluid deficit (a 1-lb weight loss equals a 500-ml fluid loss)
    c. Monitor vital signs to detect increased pulse or decreased blood pressure
    d. Assess skin turgor by evaluating resilience and resistance on the forehead or the shoulders; easily pinched skin in these locations may indicate volume deficit. (The extremities are not as useful for assessing skin turgor because of skin changes that normally occur with aging and disease conditions)
    e. Assess oral mucous membranes; sticky mucous membranes and a dry tongue may indicate fluid volume loss
    f. Monitor the results of laboratory studies—particularly BUN and hematocrit levels, which may increase in volume deficit
    g. Assess LOC; altered LOC may occur in severe volume deficit
    h. Adminster fluid replacement as indicated and as ordered. Fluid replacement should match the type of loss: I.V. fluids may be indicated for moderate or severe fluid deficits; oral fluids, for mild deficits
    i. Monitor parenteral fluid administration; when one imbalance is treated, the opposite imbalance may occur as a result of therapy
    j. Provide frequent oral care to prevent breakdown of dry mucous membranes
    k. Turn the patient at least every 2 hours to prevent skin breakdown, a problem of particular concern for a patient with volume deficit

C. Extracellular fluid volume excess (isotonic fluid volume excess)
1. General information
    a. ECF volume excess, also termed *overhydration*, results from relatively equal gains of Na and water in the ECF
    b. Osmolality is not significantly affected, because fluid and solute gains occur in equal proportions
    c. As excessive isotonic fluid accumulates in the ECF, fluid shifts into the interstitial space, resulting in edema
2. Etiology
    a. Iatrogenic overinfusion of parenteral fluids, particularly 0.9% sodium chloride (NaCl)
    b. Administration of hypertonic parenteral fluids, such as 3% or 5% NaCl
    c. Excessive ingestion of solutes, such as Na, in foods or medications
    d. Excessive administration of saline solution enemas
    e. Corticosteroid administration
    f. Congestive heart failure
    g. Chronic renal failure, with accumulation of fluid and solutes between dialysis treatments
    h. Chronic liver disease

      i. Hypoalbuminemia, which may be associated with renal disease or malnutrition

3. Clinical manifestations
    a. Acute weight gain
    b. Distended neck veins
    c. Polyuria (with normal renal function)
    d. Elevated blood pressure
    e. Full, bounding pulse
    f. Crackles auscultated in lung fields
    g. Dyspnea
    h. Tachypnea
    i. Ascites
    j. Peripheral edema

4. Diagnostic findings
    a. Decreased hematocrit (resulting from hemodilution)
    b. Normal serum sodium level
    c. Abnormal chest X-ray indicating fluid accumulation (for example, pulmonary edema or pleural effusions)

5. Nursing implications
    a. Monitor fluid intake and output for indications of excess
    b. Monitor daily weight for increases that may indicate fluid excess; keep in mind that 1 lb of weight gain equals 500-ml of fluid gain
    c. Monitor cardiopulmonary status; assess for increased blood pressure and respiratory rate
    d. Auscultate lung sounds; note crackles that do not clear with coughing, which may indicate fluid retention
    e. Assess for subjective complaints of dyspnea, such as complaints of shortness of breath or exertional dyspnea
    f. Monitor chest X-ray results to detect changes pointing to fluid accumulation
    g. Monitor laboratory study results for decreased BUN and hematocrit levels
    h. Assess for presence and amount of peripheral edema
    i. Inspect the patient confined to bed rest for sacral edema (this may be the only place that fluid accumulates in the supine position)
    j. Make sure the patient turns at least every 2 hours; edematous skin is more prone to breakdown
    k. Monitor infusion of parenteral fluids, if ordered; check the rate every hour and use I.V. controllers (pumps) as necessary to prevent fluid overload
    l. Monitor the therapeutic and adverse effects of prescribed medications—especially those which may potentiate the imbalance
    m. Teach the patient and family to monitor and record fluid intake and output and daily weight
    n. Teach the patient and family about the effects of sodium intake on fluid balance, and which food and fluids to avoid

o. Teach the patient and family how to safely administer prescribed medications

D. Intracellular fluid volume excess (hypotonic or hypo-osmotic fluid volume excess)
  1. General information
     a. ICF volume excess results from a disproportionately high loss of Na in relation to water in the ECF
     b. Na loss occurs initially from the ECF, leaving the ECF hypotonic. As a result, solute moves from the ICF into the ECF, creating a hypotonic fluid excess in the ICF
     c. ICF volume excess also may result from an increase in solute-free fluid in the ECF—for example, from overadministration of dextrose 5% in water
     d. ICF volume excess should be considered as hyponatremia because Na is the primary ECF ion and the clinical manifestations are essentially the same
     e. Osmotic changes result from a disproportionately low concentration of Na in relation to water; serum osmolality decreases to below 285 mOsm/liter
     f. Accumulation of hypo-osmotic fluid in the ICF results in a "central" intracellular edema
     g. Intracellular edema causes increased intracranial pressure, which produces the primary signs and symptoms related to the central nervous system (CNS) such as confusion and disorientation
  2. Etiology
     a. Prolonged diuretic therapy with low salt intake
     b. Replacement of lost body fluids (as from severe diaphoresis or hemorrhage) with only water or other Na-free fluids
     c. Excessive water intake linked to psychological disturbance
     d. Nasogastric (NG) tube irrigation with tap water
     e. Excessive amounts of ice chips given to patients with NG tubes or to patients who are vomiting
     f. Excessive release of antidiuretic hormone (ADH) caused by stress, surgery, trauma, or narcotic use
     g. Excessive I.V. administration of hypotonic fluids
     h. Excessive administration of tap water enemas
     i. Congestive heart failure
     j. Oat cell carcinoma of the lung, which may be associated with syndrome of inappropriate ADH secretion (SIADH)
     k. Prolonged use of oral hypoglycemic agents
     l. Prolonged use of tricyclic antidepressants
     m. Alcoholism
  3. Clinical manifestations
     a. Confusion and disorientation
     b. Muscle twitching
     c. Hyperirritability

      d. Mental disturbances, such as personality changes
      e. Headache
      f. Nausea and vomiting
      g. Convulsions
      h. Coma
      i. Polyuria in patients with healthy kidneys; oliguria in patients with renal disease
   4. Diagnostic findings
      a. Serum Na level < 120 mEq/liter
      b. Serum osmolality < 285 mOsm/liter
      c. Hypoproteinemia
   5. Nursing implications
      a. Monitor intake and output for indications of fluid excess
      b. Obtain daily weight to assess for fluid excess; remember that 1 kg of weight gain equals 1 liter of fluid gain
      c. Monitor vital signs for changes pointing to fluid excess
      d. Assess LOC and mental status for changes in cognitive function, orientation, or personality
      e. Restrict fluids, as ordered
      f. If parenteral fluid administration is ordered, monitor infusion carefully to ensure a patent I.V. line and an accurate infusion rate
      g. Administer hypotonic parenteral fluid carefully; changes in output related to weight and correlated with CNS manifestations may prevent the development of hypo-osmotic conditions
      h. Monitor laboratory study results for decreasing serum Na level and serum osmolality

E. Intracellular fluid volume deficit (hypertonic or hyperosmotic fluid volume deficit)
   1. General information
      a. ICF volume deficit results from a disproportionately high loss of water in relation to Na in the ECF
      b. Excessive water loss from the ECF leaves the ECF hypertonic. As a result, water moves from the ICF into the ECF, creating a hypertonic fluid deficit in the ICF
      c. ICF volume deficit should be considered hypernatremia because Na is the primary ion affected
      d. The osmolality of the ICF and the ECF eventually reaches an equilibrium, creating hypertonicity of both compartments when water has been lost without a corresponding solute loss
      e. Serum osmolality increases because of this hypertonicity
   2. Etiology
      a. Excessive insensible water losses, as from tachypnea, hyperventilation, hypothermia, or severe diaphoresis
      b. Decreased water intake, as from dysphagia, debilitating conditions, stroke, or coma

    c. Prolonged nothing-by-mouth (NPO) status without adequate parenteral fluid replacement

    d. Excessive administration of hypertonic fluids

    e. Excessive administration of sodium bicarbonate to treat metabolic acidosis

    f. Administration of tube feedings inadequately diluted with water

    g. Prolonged total parenteral nutrition therapy

    h. Hyperglycemia

    i. Severe gastroenteritis or diarrhea

3. Clinical manifestations

    a. Weakness

    b. Restlessness

    c. Delirium

    d. Tetany

    e. Hyperventilation

    f. Thirst

    g. Irritability

    h. Fever

    i. Flushed skin

    j. Oliguria

    k. Hyperactive deep tendon reflexes

    l. Grand mal seizures

4. Diagnostic findings

    a. Serum Na level >145 mEq/liter

    b. Serum osmolality >300 mOsm/liter

    c. Moderately high to normal hematocrit

    d. Urine specific gravity >1.030

5. Nursing implications

    a. Administer fluids as ordered—usually hypotonic I.V. fluids through a volume control device—to restore osmolality and lower serum sodium levels

    b. Monitor fluid intake and output for decreased output

    c. Obtain daily weight to distinguish weight loss from fluid loss

    d. Monitor LOC for changes that may result from too-rapid infusion of hypotonic fluid

    e. Monitor serum sodium level and serum osmolality

    f. Assess patients who are NPO for surgery or diagnostic studies for signs and symptoms of water loss

    g. Dilute tube feedings with adequate amounts of water to prevent administration of hypertonic fluids

F. Third-space fluid shifting

1. General information

    a. *Third-space fluid shifting* describes fluid accumulation in an abnormal compartment (one other than the ECF or the ICF)

    b. Creation of a "third space" requires a cellular membrane that allows water and fluid to enter but not exit

    c. Water and electrolytes in a third space are not available to maintain normal body fluid compartments, which creates solute and water imbalances

    d. Accumulation of third-space fluids usually involves swelling from inflammation with concurrent loss of fluids

    e. Some third-space fluids result from osmotic changes caused by loss of protein—for example, ascites associated with urinary protein loss

    f. Third-space fluid eventually may be reabsorbed or must be removed mechanically by such procedures as paracentesis or thoracentesis

2. Etiology

    a. Acute bowel obstruction

    b. Ascites

    c. Hypoalbuminemia

    d. Pleural effusion

    e. Acute peritonitis

    f. Burns

    g. Pancreatitis

3. Clinical manifestations

    a. Hyponatremia

    b. Tachycardia

    c. Hypotension

    d. Oliguria, with urine output <30 ml/hour

    e. Low central venous pressure

    f. Poor skin and tongue turgor

    g. Weight changes (usually gains)

4. Diagnostic findings

    a. Elevated urine specific gravity

    b. Elevated serum hematocrit

5. Nursing implications

    a. Keep in mind that third-space fluid shifting is an acute and serious problem

    b. Monitor and document the following to assess the extent and severity of the third-space shift: pulse rate and rhythm, blood pressure, respiratory rate, fluid intake and output, daily weight, and urine specific gravity and osmolality

    c. Remember that monitoring these values will also assist in estimating fluid movement changes from the third space back to normal fluid compartments

    d. Keep in mind that parenteral fluid administration will provide symptomatic relief but will not resolve the problem; rather, it will increase the patient's total body weight without making the third-space fluid available to the body

    e. Be aware that correction may require surgery or may occur spontaneously as a physiologic shift that can be predicted to occur within 48 to 72 hours

G. Patients at risk for water imbalances
1. General information
   a. Certain disease states, medication use, and age are factors influencing a person's susceptibility to water imbalances
   b. These factors affect the routes of water gains or losses, homeostatic regulatory systems, or the body's ability to compensate for imbalances
   c. The three groups of patients most at risk are infants and children (because of the immaturity of their regulatory mechanisms and physiologic differences in body composition), older adults (because of physiologic changes, decreased access from compromised mobility, and diminished compensatory reserves), and chronically ill patients (because of increased physiologic stress and diminished compensatory reserves)
2. Newborns, infants, and children
   a. In newborns, water constitutes 80% of total body weight (90% in premature newborns)
   b. In infants, about 40% of body water is in the ECF, compared to 20% in adults
   c. By age 2, a child's percentage of total body weight as water approaches 50%, as in an adult
   d. An infant may exchange 50% of the ECF daily, compared with 18% in an adult
   e. The immature kidneys concentrate urine inefficiently and, combined with the previous factors, contribute to the potential for rapid dehydration in disease states
   f. Compared with adults, who may be able to tolerate fluid imbalances for days, infants and young children can develop an acute imbalance in hours
   g. Because the ratio of body surface area to weight is several times greater in infants and children than in adults, infants and children are at greater risk for fluid imbalance from insensible water loss through the skin
   h. Because infants and children have a relatively greater GI tract surface area, they can experience greater water losses there
3. Older adults
   a. After age 65, the percentage of total body water progressively decreases to between 40% and 50%
   b. Progressively decreasing renal function impairs excretion of heavy solute loads, such as those from tube feedings
   c. Risk of hyperglycemia and osmotic diuresis increases because of decreased pancreatic functioning and glucose tolerance
   d. Cardiovascular function deterioration impairs compensation for hypotensive states
   e. Decreased mobility and cognition may compromise consumption of adequate fluids (and foods), particularly during illness

    f. Diminished thirst mechanism increases the risk of dehydration, especially in hot weather

    g. Diminished renal function increases the risk of water imbalance from certain medications—particularly diuretics and electrolyte replacement supplements

    h. Decreased skin elasticity makes skin turgor a poor indicator of hydration status

4. Chronically ill patients

    a. Illness affecting major body systems may compromise changes in fluid balance

    b. Diabetes and other endocrine diseases indirectly affect fluid balance

    c. Patients with renal insufficiency or chronic renal failure must maintain proper fluid balance to prevent acute illness

Points to Remember

Volume (or isotonic) imbalances primarily affect the extracellular fluid (ECF) and involve relatively equal losses or gains of sodium and water.

Osmotic imbalances primarily affect the intracellular fluid (ICF) and involve relatively unequal losses or gains of sodium and water.

Peripheral edema results from the accumulation of water in the ECF.

Third-space shifting involves fluid accumulation in an abnormal compartment (one other than the ECF or the ICF).

Those at greatest risk for water imbalances are infants and children, older adults, and chronically ill patients.

Glossary

Hypertonic—having a higher solute concentration than another solution

Hypotonic—having a lower solute concentration than another solution

Isotonic—having the same solute concentration as another solution, such as normal body fluids

Third space—an abnormal compartment created by a change in the normal cellular membrane caused by trauma, edema, or manipulation for example, abcess, ascites or burns

Electrolyte Imbalances

Learning Objectives

After studying this section, the reader should be able to:

- State laboratory test values representative of each electrolyte imbalance.

- List the clinical manifestations of each electrolyte imbalance.

- Describe the nursing implications for a patient with each electrolyte imbalance.

- Identify the ECG changes that occur with potassium, calcium, and magnesium imbalances.

- Describe those patients at greatest risk for electrolyte imbalances.

VI. Electrolyte Imbalances

A. Introduction
1. Electrolyte imbalances are common in patients requiring nursing care
2. Certain electrolyte imbalances, such as those involving sodium (Na), develop gradually and usually are not life-threatening
3. Other electrolyte imbalances, such as those involving potassium (K), can quickly become life-threatening and possibly fatal if not recognized and treated promptly
4. Changes in serum concentrations of chloride (Cl) alone rarely cause problems; chloride can be depleted by diuretics, especially furosemide; imbalances usually are reflected as metabolic acid-base imbalances (See "Metabolic acidosis" and "Metabolic alkalosis" in Section VII, and Appendix B: *Selected Laboratory Tests,* pages 111-112)

B. Sodium deficit: hyponatremia
1. General information
   a. Hyponatremia begins with an excessive Na loss or an excessive water gain in the extracellular fluid (ECF)
   b. As ECF osmolality decreases from Na deficiency or water excess, Na moves out of the intracellular fluid (ICF) into the ECF, and water moves into the ICF, which alters ICF osmolality
   c. Water movement into the ICF causes cellular swelling and, eventually, central nervous system (CNS) changes
   d. Hyponatremia may result from increased Na and water levels in the ECF with a relatively greater water increase, as in congestive heart failure, liver failure, and nephrotic syndrome
   e. Hyponatremia may result from decreased Na and water levels in the ECF with a relatively greater Na decrease
2. Etiology
   a. Prolonged diuretic therapy
   b. Excessive diaphoresis
   c. Insufficient Na intake
   d. Excessive Na loss from trauma, such as massive burns
   e. Severe GI fluid losses from gastric suctioning or lavage, prolonged vomiting or diarrhea, or laxative abuse
   f. Administration of hypotonic fluids
   g. Compulsive water drinking linked to a psychological disturbance
   h. Labor induction with oxytocin
   i. Adrenal insufficiency
   j. Sodium-losing renal disease
   k. Cystic fibrosis
   l. Alcoholism
   m. SIADH

3. Clinical manifestations
   a. Headache
   b. Faintness
   c. Confusion
   d. Muscle cramps
   e. Muscle twitching
   f. Normal or increased weight
   g. Convulsions
   h. Coma
4. Diagnostic findings
   a. Serum Na level <136 mEq/liter
   b. Urine specific gravity <1.010 (>1.012 in SIADH)
   c. Serum osmolality <285 mOsm/kg
5. Nursing implications
   a. Monitor and record fluid intake and output; relatively greater increases in water in relation to Na will decrease output in relation to intake
   b. Restrict fluid intake, as ordered; this is the primary treatment for hyponatremia
   c. Administer parenteral fluids, as ordered; Na should be administered sparingly to prevent increases in total fluid volume
   d. Monitor and record vital signs, particularly blood pressure and pulse rate
   e. Assess skin integrity at least every 8 hours
   f. Administer I.V. isotonic or hypertonic saline solutions cautiously to avoid inducing hypernatremia from excessive or too-rapid infusion
   g. Monitor serum Na levels to determine treatment effectiveness
   h. Teach the patient and family to use diuretics carefully to avoid excessive Na loss
   i. Monitor daily weight for increases linked to water excess
   j. Teach the patient and family to follow any sodium-restricted diet carefully to ensure low, but still adequate, Na intake

C. Sodium excess: hypernatremia
1. General information
   a. Increased serum Na levels usually indicate a water deficit in the ECF, which moves water out of the ICF to equilibrate
   b. Cellular shrinkage results from increased Na levels in the ECF, increasing serum osmolality and water movement water from the ICF into the ECF
   c. Cellular shrinkage in the CNS causes impaired neurologic and cognitive function
   d. Hypernatremia usually results in ICF volume deficit
2. Etiology
   a. Significantly deficient water intake
   b. Hypertonic parenteral fluid administration
   c. Hypertonic tube feedings
   d. Excessive salt ingestion

  e. Severe watery diarrhea or severe insensible water losses, as from heat stroke or prolonged high fever

  f. Major burns

  g. Use of inadequately diluted baby formulas

  h. Use of high-protein liquid diets without adequate fluid intake

  i. Osmotic diuresis, as in hyperosmolar hyperglycemic nonketotic coma (HHNC)

  j. Diabetes insipidus

3. Clinical manifestations

  a. Extreme thirst

  b. Tachycardia

  c. Low-grade fever

  d. Dry, sticky tongue and oral mucosa

  e. Disorientation

  f. Hallucinations

  g. Lethargy progressing to coma

  h. Hyperactive deep tendon reflexes

  i. Seizures

  j. Coma

4. Diagnostic findings

  a. Serum Na level >145 mEq/liter

  b. Urine specific gravity > 1.015

  c. Serum osmolality >295 mOsm/kg

5. Nursing implications

  a. Monitor and record fluid intake and output; the patient may have seriously decreased output

  b. Monitor daily weight for changes

  c. Assess for changes in mental function and level of consciousness

  d. Monitor and record vital signs, particularly blood pressure, pulse rate, and temperature

  e. Cautiously administer ordered parenteral fluids (usually hypotonic Na solution or any hypotonic solution except D_5W) to prevent fluid overload and resultant cerebral edema

  f. Assess skin and mucous membranes for signs of breakdown and infection

  g. Provide thorough oral hygiene to keep mucous membranes moist and to decrease odor

  h. Monitor laboratory test results for trends pointing to hypernatremia

  i. Ensure adequate water administration when a patient is receiving hypertonic fluids, to prevent solute overload; for example, dilute tube feedings, and infuse total parenteral nutrition at the prescribed rate

  j. Teach the patient and family about foods and over-the-counter medications high in Na, to prevent accidental overingestion of Na

  k. Encourage the patient and family to minimize use of Na in cooking and at the table

  l. If necessary, instruct the patient and family about sodium-restricted diets to promote compliance

D. Potassium deficit: hypokalemia
 1. General information
    a. Hypokalemia usually results from excessive excretion or inadequate intake of K
    b. K functions as the major intracellular cation and balances Na in the ECF to maintain the electroneutrality of body fluids
    c. K is freely excreted by the kidneys and is not stored by the body
    d. About 40 mEq of K is excreted in 1 liter of urine
    e. K is also exchanged for the hydrogen ion when changes in the body's acid-base balance indicate a need for cation exchange; K moves into the cells in exchange for hydrogen
    f. Increased cellular uptake of K occurs in insulin excess, alkalosis, and certain disorders, such as renal failure
 2. Etiology
    a. Prolonged diuretic therapy (for example, with thiazides or furosemide)
    b. Inadequate dietary K intake
    c. Administration of K-deficient parenteral fluids
    d. Severe diaphoresis
    e. Severe GI fluid losses from gastric suctioning or lavage, prolonged vomiting or diarrhea, or laxative abuse without K replacement
    f. Excessive secretion of endogenous insulin or administration of exogenous insulin
    g. Excessive stress (corticosteroid release results in Na retention and K excretion)
    h. Alkalosis
    i. Hepatic disease
    j. Hyperaldosteronism
    k. Renal tubular defect (tubular acidosis)
    l. Acute alcoholism
 3. Clinical manifestations
    a. Anorexia
    b. Nausea and vomiting
    c. Drowsiness, lethargy
    d. Leg cramps
    e. Muscle weakness, especially in the legs
    f. Hyporeflexia
    g. Paresthesias
    h. Decreased bowel motility (ileus)
    i. Hypotension
    j. Cardiac dysrhythmias, such as premature atrial contractions or premature ventricular contractions
    k. Paresthesia
    l. Coma
 4. Diagnostic findings
    a. ECG changes: ST segment depression, flattened T waves, U waves present or superimposed on the T waves

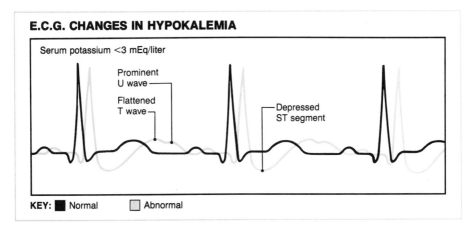

E.C.G. CHANGES IN HYPOKALEMIA

Serum potassium <3 mEq/liter

Prominent U wave

Flattened T wave

Depressed ST segment

KEY: ■ Normal ☐ Abnormal

b. Serum K level <3.5 mEq/liter
c. Elevated pH and bicarbonate level
d. Urine specific gravity <1.010
e. Slightly elevated serum glucose level

5. Nursing implications
   a. Monitor for signs and symptoms of hypokalemia in patients who are at risk
   b. Be aware that patients receiving diuretics are more susceptible to hypokalemia and require close observation; patients receiving digitalis are in danger if hypokalemia occurs because hypokalemia and digitalis cause digitalis toxicity
   c. Monitor fluid intake and output closely; because 40 mEq of K is lost per liter of urine output, diuresis puts the patient at risk for serious K loss
   d. Administer oral K replacements in at least 4 oz of fluid or with food to prevent gastric irritation
   e. Administer I.V. K supplement infusions cautiously, always diluted and mixed thoroughly in adequate amounts of fluid; such patients should be placed on a cardiac monitor.
   f. Never administer K through I.V. push or as a bolus, which could prove fatal
   g. Assess the I.V. infusion site for signs and symptoms of infiltration or pain; high-concentration solutions may cause discomfort and irritation
   h. Monitor heart rate, rhythm, and ECG tracings in a severely hypokalemic patient with a serum K level <3 mEq/liter; in a patient receiving >5 mEq of K per hour I.V.; and in a patient receiving I.V. K at a concentration >40 mEq K to 1 liter of fluid
   i. Monitor vital signs, particularly pulse rate and blood pressure; postural hypotension may occur with hypokalemia
   j. Monitor serum K levels carefully; keep in mind that relatively minor changes in serum K levels can cause serious cardiac complications

    k. Monitor for signs of metabolic alkalosis, such as irritability and confusion, which may be linked to hypokalemia

    l. Teach the patient and family measures to increase dietary intake of K, especially if the patient is taking a diuretic

    m. Instruct the patient and family in how to properly use oral K supplements

E. Potassium excess: hyperkalemia
1. General information
    a. Hyperkalemia results from impaired renal excretion of K or excessive K intake
    b. Hyperkalemia can also occur in metabolic acidosis; K moves into serum as hydrogen (H) moves into cells, lowering the pH
    c. Acidosis-associated hyperkalemia involves a movement of K from cells into serum, rather than an increase in total body K levels
    d. Excessive serum K levels act as a myocardial depressant, causing decreased heart rate, decreased cardiac output, and possible cardiac arrest
    e. Hyperkalemia causes skeletal muscle weakness, usually the initial symptom that causes patients to seek health care assistance
    f. Hyperkalemia also causes smooth muscle hyperactivity, particularly in the GI tract, which can result in colic and diarrhea
2. Etiology
    a. Increased dietary K intake, especially with decreased urine output
    b. Excessive administration of K supplements
    c. Excessive use of salt substitutes, most of which use some form of K as a substitute for Na
    d. Use of K-sparing diuretics, such as spironolactone
    e. Severe, widespread cell damage, as from burns, trauma, crush injuries, intravascular hemolysis, or increased catabolism
    f. Administration of large volumes of blood that is nearing the expiration date ("old" blood undergoes increased cell hemolysis, resulting in the release of K as cells die)
    g. Lysis of tumor cells from chemotherapy (K is released from dying cells into the ECF)
    h. Hyponatremia
    i. Hypoaldosteronism
    j. Metabolic acidosis
    k. Acute or chronic renal failure
3. Clinical manifestations
    a. Apathy
    b. Confusion
    c. Paresthesias and numbness in extremities
    d. Abdominal cramps
    e. Nausea
    f. Flaccid muscle paralysis
    g. Diarrhea

      h. Oliguria
      i. Bradycardia
      j. Idioventricular cardiac dysrhythmias
      k. Cardiac arrest
  4. Diagnostic findings
      a. Serum K level > 5.5 mEq/liter
      b. Decreased arterial pH
      c. ECG abnormalities: tall, tented T waves; wide QRS complex; prolonged PR interval; depressed ST segment; flattened or absent P wave (if not reversed, can lead to asystole)

E.C.G. CHANGES IN HYPERKALEMIA

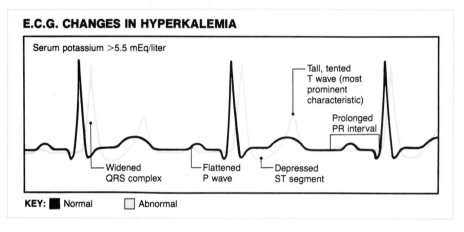

Serum potassium >5.5 mEq/liter

Tall, tented T wave (most prominent characteristic)

Prolonged PR interval

Widened QRS complex

Flattened P wave

Depressed ST segment

KEY: ■ Normal   ☐ Abnormal

  5. Nursing implications
      a. Monitor patients at risk for hyperkalemia, specifically those in acidosis and those receiving K or K-sparing diuretics
      b. Before administering I.V. K supplements, determine whether the patient has a urine output > 30 ml/hour; inability to adequately excrete K may lead to dangerously high K levels
      c. Remember, cardiac monitoring and a 12-lead ECG are indicated with elevated serum K levels; a patient with ECG changes may need aggressive treatment to prevent cardiac arrest. The term "symptomatic" hyperkalemia refers to ECG changes that are present with a serum K level > 5.5 mEq/liter
      d. Assess cardiovascular status by monitoring pulse rate and rhythm and blood pressure; blood pressure may be elevated initially but may drop as cardiac changes occur, and pulse rate may be slow and regular or irregular, or fast and irregular
      e. Assess for hyperactive bowel sounds and diarrhea
      f. Monitor serum K levels to determine treatment effectiveness
      g. Assess motor and sensory function, especially of the extremities, for changes that may indicate changes in serum K levels
      h. Monitor neurologic status for changes; loss of consciousness may not occur with severe hyperkalemia until cardiac arrest occurs

    i. Be prepared to give calcium gluconate by slow I.V. infusion in acute cases to counteract the myocardial depressant effects of hyperkalemia; the patient must be on a cardiac monitor during administration

    j. Keep in mind that symptomatic acute hyperkalemia may be treated temporarily on an emergency basis by administering dextrose 50% and regular insulin I.V. to facilitate K movement back into the cells

    k. Prepare the patient for the possibility of dialysis, either peritoneal or hemodialysis, which may be ordered in acute cases (in acute symptomatic hyperkalemia, only hemodialysis is used)

    l. As ordered, administer sodium polystyrene sulfonate (Kayexalate)—a cation-exchange resin—orally or rectally to decrease serum K levels as the K moves into the bowel space and the Na moves into the bowel cell

    m. Administer oral sodium polystyrene sulfonate with sorbitol or another osmotic substance to enhance its K-removing action

    n. Be aware that oral sodium polystyrene sulfonate should be excreted within 24 hours to prevent bowel perforation; administer soapsuds enemas as necessary to promote excretion

    o. Administer rectal sodium polystyrene sulfonate as a retention enema; patients commonly experience cramps or diarrhea, making enema administration and retention difficult; use of an indwelling urinary drainage catheter with the balloon inflated helps with enema administration and retention

    p. Monitor for signs of hypernatremia and congestive heart failure in a patient receiving sodium polystyrene sulfonate

    q. Administer sodium bicarbonate, as ordered, to a patient with acidosis to decrease serum K levels by creating alkalosis

    r. Teach patients, particularly those with renal failure or renal insufficiency, about foods and fluids high in K and the importance of avoiding them to prevent hyperkalemia

    s. Remind patients that most salt substitutes are high in K

    t. Be aware that hemolysis of blood samples, either from too tight a tourniquet or too rapid pulling of blood into a vial or syringe, may cause falsely elevated K levels (pseudohyperkalemia); a sample should be redrawn if no clinical symptoms exist

F. Calcium deficit: hypocalcemia

  1. General information

    a. Hypocalcemia results from abnormalities of parathyroid hormone secretion or from inadequate dietary intake or excessive losses of bound, ionized (unbound), or total body calcium (Ca)

    b. Hypocalcemia usually reflects decreased circulating ionized Ca levels

    c. Hypocalcemia can cause skeletal and neuromuscular abnormalities

    d. Hypocalcemia impairs clotting mechanisms

    e. Because Ca helps maintain cellular integrity, hypocalcemia affects cell membrane integrity and permeability

    f. Because half of ingested Ca is bound to protein, serum protein abnormalities influence serum Ca levels

    g. Because half of ionized Ca is absorbed in the gut with vitamin D, GI

tract or vitamin D abnormalities decrease serum Ca levels
   h. Symptoms of hypocalcemia reflect increased neural excitability and
      spontaneous stimulation of sensory and motor fibers
2. Etiology
   a. Surgically induced or primary hypoparathyroidism
   b. Acute or chronic renal failure
   c. Chronic malabsorption syndrome
   d. Vitamin D deficiency
   e. Inadequate exposure to ultraviolet light
   f. Chronic insufficient dietary intake of Ca
   g. Hyperphosphatemia
   h. Acute pancreatitis
   i. Administration of large amounts of citrated blood
   j. Alkalosis
   k. Hypoalbuminemia
   l. Hypomagnesemia
3. Clinical manifestations
   a. Muscle cramps or tremors
   b. Hyperactive deep tendon reflexes
   c. Paresthesias of the fingers, toes, and face
   d. Tetany
   e. Positive Trousseau's sign
   f. Positive Chvostek's sign
   g. Spasm of laryngeal and bronchial muscles
   h. Spasm of abdominal muscles
   i. Confusion
   k. Moodiness and anxiety
   l. Memory loss
   m. Seizures
   n. Dysrhythmias
4. Diagnostic findings
   a. ECG: prolonged QT interval and ST segment

E.C.G. CHANGES IN HYPOCALCEMIA

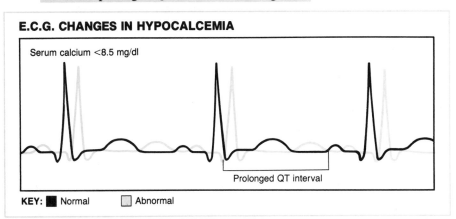

Serum calcium <8.5 mg/dl

Prolonged QT interval

KEY: ■ Normal   ☐ Abnormal

    b. Serum Ca level <8.5 mg/dl

    c. Ionized Ca level <50%

    d. Light precipitation on Sulkowitch's urine test

    e. Prolonged prothrombin time and partial thromboplastin time

5. Nursing implications

    a. Carefully assess patients at increased risk for hypocalcemia, especially after parathyroidectomy or massive transfusions

    b. Remember, seizure precautions, may be indicated based on the extent of musculoskeletal complications

    c. Institute safety precautions, such as padded bed rails and restraints, to prevent injury, especially if the patient is confused

    d. Remember, Ca may be given initially as a slow I.V. bolus, followed by a slow I.V. drip infusion if Ca deficit is acute

    e. Administer I.V. Ca replacements carefully, ensuring that the vein is patent; infiltration can cause tissue necrosis and sloughing

    f. Place the patient on a cardiac monitor and observe for changes in heart rate and rhythm

    g. Monitor a patient receiving I.V. Ca for dysrhythmias, especially if he is also taking digitalis (Ca sensitizes the heart to digitalis); too-rapid administration can lead to cardiac arrest; I.V. Ca may be contraindicated in patients receiving digitalis

    h. Expect to administer oral Ca supplements or vitamin D for mild to moderate hypocalcemia

    i. Assess the patient's nutritional intake for Ca or vitamin D deficiencies; adjust dietary intake to increase Ca

    j. Keep calcium gluconate at the bedside of a patient recovering from parathyroid or thyroid surgery, for administration if a rapid drop in serum Ca level occurs

    k. Teach the patient and family about foods and fluids high in calcium, such as dairy products and green, leafy vegetables

    l. Teach the patient and family that exercise enhances Ca mobilization from bone to replenish ECF levels

    m. Teach the patient and family that female hormones, such as estrogen, may be administered to maintain adequate Ca levels in patients with osteoporosis

G. Calcium excess: hypercalcemia

1. General information

    a. Hypercalcemia occurs when the rate of Ca entry into the ECF exceeds the rate of renal Ca excretion

    b. Normally, bone resorption and formation occur at the same rate; mobilization of Ca from bone, for any reason, results in increased serum Ca levels

    c. Increased intestinal absorption of Ca—from either increased availability, increased vitamin D absorption, or altered GI metabolism—also results in increased serum Ca levels

    d. Renal abnormalities (particularly of the tubules) that interfere with secretion and excretion of Ca also can cause increased serum Ca levels

    e. Hypercalcemia symptoms are directly related to the degree of serum Ca elevation; severe symptoms may occur with levels >16 mg/dl

    f. Patients with metastatic cancer are at especially high risk for hypercalcemia

2. Etiology

    a. Excessive intake of Ca supplements

    b. Excessive use of Ca-containing antacids (phosphate-binding gels)

    c. Prolonged immobility

    d. Excessive vitamin D intake

    e. Use of thiazide diuretics

    f. Primary hyperparathyroidism

    g. Metastatic carcinoma

    h. Thyrotoxicosis

    i. Hypophosphatemia

    j. Renal tubular acidosis

3. Clinical manifestations

    a. Muscle weakness or flaccidity

    b. Personality changes, such as neurotic behavior progressing to psychoses

    c. Nausea and vomiting

    d. Extreme thirst

    e. Anorexia

    f. Constipation

    g. Polyuria

    h. Urinary calculi

    i. Pathologic fractures

    j. Metastatic calcifications, particularly in the cornea and skin (causes itching)

    k. Dysrhythmias and cardiac arrest

    l. Altered level of consciousness

    m. Coma

4. Diagnostic findings

    a. Serum Ca level >10.5 mg/dl

    b. Bone changes on X-ray, such as pathologic fractures

    c. Dense precipitation on Sulkowitch's urine test

    d. ECG changes: possible prolonged QT interval and ST segment

5. Nursing implications

    a. Monitor patients at risk for hypercalcemia, especially those with hyperparathyroidism or cancer and those on long-term bed rest

    b. Ambulate the patient as soon as possible to prevent Ca mobilization from the bone

    c. Have the patient drink 3 to 4 liters of fluids daily (if not contraindicated) to stimulate renal Ca excretion

    d. Offer the patient foods or fluids high in Na (if not contraindicated), because the kidneys excrete Ca in favor of Na

E.C.G. CHANGES IN HYPERCALCEMIA

Serum calcium >10.5 mg/dl

Shortened QT interval

KEY: ■ Normal   □ Abnormal

  e. In a patient with acute moderate to severe hypercalcemia (levels >13 mg/dl), administer I.V. isotonic normal saline solution, usually at a rate of 200 to 500 ml/hour, to reverse dehydration and promote urinary Ca excretion
  f. Administer loop diuretics, such as furosemide, to prevent volume overload with I.V. normal saline solution and to increase urinary Ca excretion
  g. Remember, calcitonin may be given to lower serum Ca levels temporarily in acute cases if I.V. normal saline solution is ineffective
  h. Place the patient on a cardiac monitor to detect dysrhythmias
  i. In patients with hypercalcemia and low serum phosphorus (P) levels, administer inorganic P salts orally, rectally, or I.V. to lower serum Ca levels by inhibiting bone resorption, reducing Ca absorption, and forming a Ca-P complex
  j. Keep in mind that corticosteroids may be used to decrease GI absorption of Ca
  k. Monitor serum Ca, P, and Na levels to determine treatment effectiveness and to detect new imbalances resulting from therapy
  l. Institute safety precautions, such as restraints and elevated side rails, for a confused and disoriented patient
  m. Teach the patient and family signs and symptoms to assess, such as personality changes, muscle weakness, and pathologic fractures
  n. Teach the patient to avoid Ca-containing foods and fluids, particularly dairy products, to prevent increased serum Ca levels

H. Phosphorus deficit: hypophosphatemia
  1. General information
    a. Hypophosphatemia commonly results from decreased intestinal absorption of P
    b. It also may result from renal wasting of P as a method of controlling acid-base balance or during diuresis

    c. Hypophosphatemia may result from P redistribution from the ECF to the ICF, as may occur from I.V. glucose administration

    d. P in the form of adenosine triphosphate (ATP) helps maintain the integrity of cell membranes and produces energy within cells

    e. P as 2,3-diphosphoglycerate functions in red blood cells to promote oxygen release to cells

    f. Serum P levels are influenced by diet, parathyroid hormone, and renal function

2. Etiology

    a. Inadequate dietary P intake

    b. Severe, prolonged vomiting

    c. Excessive administration of P-binding gels

    d. Thiazide diuretic therapy

    e. Alcoholism and alcohol withdrawal

    f. Adminstration of carbohydrates or total parenteral nutrition (TPN) without P to malnourished patients

    g. I.V. glucose or insulin administration (moves P into skeletal muscle, decreasing serum levels)

    h. Malabsorption syndromes

    i. Hyperparathyroidism

    j. Severe metabolic acidosis, such as in diabetic ketoacidosis

    k. Respiratory alkalosis

    l. Thermal burns

    m. Hypokalemia

    n. Hypomagnesemia

    o. Acute gout

    p. Aldosteronism

3. Clinical manifestations

    a. Paresthesias

    b. Profound muscle weakness

    c. Muscle pain and tenderness

    d. Anorexia

    e. Malaise

    f. Rapid, shallow respirations

    g. Altered level of consciousness

    h. Seizures

    i. Nystagmus, unequal pupils

    j. Heart failure

    k. Hemolytic anemia

    l. Platelet dysfunction

4. Diagnostic findings

    a. Serum P level <3 mg/dl

    b. Hypercalciuria

    c. Elevated creatine phosphokinase (CPK) levels when serum P levels are < 1 mg/dl for a day or more

5. Nursing implications
   a. Monitor patients at risk for hypophosphatemia, especially those receiving TPN without P replacement
   b. Assess for paresthesias, particularly in the circumoral area—an early sign of hypophosphatemia
   c. Initiate safety precautions for a patient with confusion or decreased level of consciousness
   d. Assess for signs and symptoms of infection; in hypophosphatemia, granulocytes have less ability to fight foreign bodies
   e. Assess a patient with hypophosphatemia for signs and symptoms of hypercalcemia, such as urinary calculi, because of the reciprocal relationship between Ca and P
   f. Expect to administer oral P supplements to a patient with mild to moderate hypophosphatemia
   g. Use caution when administering parenteral P to a patient with severe hypophosphatemia; hypocalcemia may occur as P levels rise
   h. Remember that malnourished patients should be refed gradually to avoid hypophosphatemia resulting from I.V. glucose administration
   i. Instruct the patient and family in measures to increase dietary P intake

I. Phosphorus excess: hyperphosphatemia

1. General information
   a. Hyperphosphatemia most commonly results from decreased P excretion in renal disease
   b. Of the remaining cases of hyperphosphatemia, about half have no explainable etiology; some cases may be attributed to increased dietary P intake
   c. Lysis of tumor cells during cancer chemotherapy can result in P redistribution from the ICF to the ECF, possibly causing hyperphosphatemia
   d. Laxatives and P-based enemas may increase P absorption from the GI tract
2. Etiology
   a. Acute or chronic renal failure
   b. Excessive dietary P intake
   c. Exessive vitamin D use
   d. Hypoparathyroidism
   e. Cancer chemotherapy
   f. Excessive use of laxatives and P-based enemas
3. Clinical manifestations
   a. Tetany
   b. Circumoral paresthesias
   c. Muscle spasms
   d. Seizures (chronic P increase may decrease Ca levels)
   e. Soft tissue calcification (with long-standing hyperphosphatemia)

4. Diagnostic findings
   a. Serum P level >4.5 mg/dl
   b. Decreased serum Ca level
5. Nursing implications
   a. Monitor patients at risk, particularly those with hypocalcemia
   b. Initiate seizure precautions in patients with elevated P levels
   c. Monitor for neuromuscular irritability, which accompanies high P levels
   d. Remember that P-binding antacids, such as aluminum hydroxide gel, may be administered to lower serum P levels
   e. Keep in mind that acetazolamide may be administered to increase urinary P excretion; dialysis can also be used for hyperphosphatemia
   f. Administer Ca supplements to promote elevation of serum Ca levels, which lowers serum P levels
   g. Teach the patient and family to avoid foods and fluids high in P, such as cheeses, nuts, whole-grain cereals, dried fruits, and vegetables
   h. Teach the patient and family to avoid excessive use of enemas and laxatives containing P

J. Magnesium deficit: hypomagnesemia
   1. General information
      a. Hypomagnesemia results from excessive magnesium (Mg) loss from increased renal excretion or GI fluid losses, insufficient dietary Mg intake, or movement of Mg from the ECF to the ICF
      b. Mg, the second most abundant intracellular cation, is essential for neuromuscular integration; hypomagnesemia increases muscle cell irritability and contractility
      c. Mg also activates enzyme systems and contributes to intracellular biochemical reactions
      d. Hypomagnesemia causes decreased blood pressure and may result in ventricular dysrhythmias
      e. Hypomagnesemia commonly is mistaken for hypokalemia, which often occurs simultaneously
   2. Etiology
      a. Excessive dietary intake of Ca or vitamin D
      b. Severe GI fluid losses from gastric suctioning or lavage, prolonged vomiting or diarrhea, or laxative abuse
      c. Prolonged, excessive diuretic therapy
      d. Administration of I.V. fluids or TPN without Mg replacement
      e. Prolonged malnutrition or starvation
      f. Malabsorption syndromes
      g. Ulcerative colitis
      h. Hypercalcemia
      i. Hypoparathyroidism
      j. Hypoaldosteronism
      k. High-dose steroid use
      l. Cancer chemotherapy

    m. Gentamicin therapy
    n. Burns and debridement therapy
    o. Sepsis
    p. Pancreatitis
    q. Diabetic ketoacidosis
    r. Chronic alcoholism and alcohol withdrawal
    s. Pregnancy-induced hypertension
3. Clinical manifestations
    a. Tachycardia and other dysrhythmias, hypotension
    b. Tremors
    c. Tetany
    d. Hyperactive deep tendon reflexes
    e. Positive Chvostek's and Trousseau's signs
    f. Memory loss
    g. Emotional lability
    h. Confusion
    i. Dizziness
    j. Anorexia
    k. Nausea
    l. Hallucinations
    m. Seizures
    n. Coma
4. Diagnostic findings
    a. Serum Mg level < 1.5 mEq/liter (clinical manifestations occur at about 1 mEq/liter)
    b. Hypocalcemia
    c. Hypokalemia
    d. ECG changes: prolonged PR and QT intervals, wide QRS complex, depressed ST segment and inverted T wave, tachydysrhythmias, including the classic ECG changes seen with digitalis toxicity

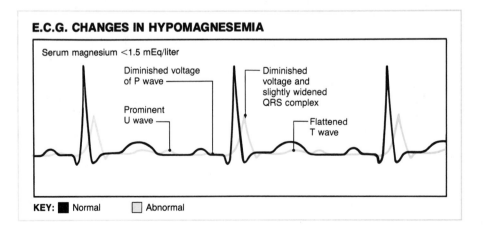

E.C.G. CHANGES IN HYPOMAGNESEMIA

Serum magnesium <1.5 mEq/liter

Diminished voltage of P wave

Prominent U wave

Diminished voltage and slightly widened QRS complex

Flattened T wave

KEY: ■ Normal ☐ Abnormal

5. Nursing implications
  a. Monitor patients at risk for hypomagnesemia, particularly those with hypokalemia and those receiving TPN without Mg replacement
  b. Monitor a patient taking digitalis for signs of digitalis toxicity, the risk of which is increased in hypomagnesemia resulting from the body's retention of digitalis
  c. Institute cardiac monitoring in a patient with severe hypomagnesemia
  d. Initiate seizure precautions to prevent patient injury
  e. Monitor for signs and symptoms of hypomagnesemia during prolonged infusion of Mg-free I.V. fluids
  f. Remember, hypomagnesemia may be treated with oral, intramuscular, or I.V. Mg salts
  g. Administer I.V. Mg slowly; too-rapid infusion can cause cardiac or respiratory arrest
  h. During I.V. Mg therapy, monitor urine output; it should be at least 100 ml every 4 hours for adequate renal Mg elimination
  i. Assess deep tendon reflexes during long-term I.V. Mg therapy; if reflexes are absent, hold the dose and notify the doctor
  j. For a patient experiencing seizures, administer a 10% Mg solution at a rate no greater than 1.5 ml/minute
  k. Monitor serum Mg and K levels to evaluate treatment effectiveness
  l. Assess for laryngeal stridor, which may indicate the onset of airway obstruction with hypomagnesemia
  m. Initiate safety precautions, such as elevated bed rails and restraints, for a confused patient
  n. Monitor for dysphagia, especially when giving medications or foods, because swallowing may be impaired
  o. Teach the patient and family about the dangers of diuretic abuse and its link to hypomagnesemia
  p. Teach the patient and family about foods high in Mg, such as green vegetables, nuts, beans, and fruits

K. Magnesium excess: hypermagnesemia
  1. General information
    a. Hypermagnesemia usually results from renal failure
    b. Excessive Mg intake commonly involves over-the-counter medications or parenteral Mg
    c. Magnesium produces a sedative effect on the neuromuscular junction, inhibits acetylcholine release, and diminishes muscle cell excitability
    d. Hypermagnesemia can cause hypotension and possibly cardiac arrest
  2. Etiology
    a. Renal failure
    b. Excessive use of Mg-containing antacids or laxatives
    c. Excessive administration of parenteral Mg
    d. Untreated diabetic ketoacidosis
    e. Hypoadrenalism

    f. Hemodialysis using hard water high in Mg
3. Clinical manifestations
    a. Lethargy and drowsiness
    b. Depressed neuromuscular activity
    c. Depressed respirations
    d. Sensation of warmth throughout the body
    e. Hypoactive deep tendon refexes
    f. Hypotension
    g. Bradycardia
    h. Cardiac arrest
    i. Coma
4. Diagnostic findings
    a. Serum Mg level > 3 mEq/liter
    b. ECG changes: prolonged PR interval, QRS complex, and QT interval; heart block; asystole

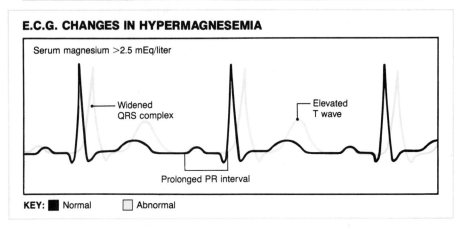

E.C.G. CHANGES IN HYPERMAGNESEMIA

Serum magnesium >2.5 mEq/liter

Widened QRS complex

Elevated T wave

Prolonged PR interval

KEY: ■ Normal   □ Abnormal

5. Nursing implications
    a. Monitor patients at risk, especially those with conditions predisposing to hypermagnesemia, such as renal failure
    b. Monitor vital signs—particularly blood pressure, which can drop precipitously, and respirations, which may be depressed and can progress to apnea
    c. Assess neuromuscular status for deficits; evaluate reflexes, grip strength, and respiratory muscle function
    d. In a patient with renal failure, check for any standing orders for Mg-containing medication, such as laxatives or antacids; administer them cautiously
    e. Institute cardiac monitoring for a patient with serum Mg levels >7 mEq/liter, who is at increased risk for cardiac arrest
    f. Be prepared to administer calcium gluconate, an Mg antagonist, to temporarily relieve symptoms in an emergency

g. Monitor serum Mg levels for changes to evaluate the patient's response to therapy

h. Teach the patient and family to minimize intake of foods high in Mg, such as green vegetables, nuts, beans, and fruits

L. Patients at risk for electrolyte imbalances

1. General information

a. Patients vary in their susceptibility to electrolyte imbalances

b. Age- and illness-related physiologic changes affect the body's ability to compensate for imbalances

c. Because of the close association between water and electrolytes, patients at risk for water imbalances are also at risk for electrolyte imbalances

d. Three groups of patients at highest risk are infants and children, older adults, and chronically ill patients

2. Infants and children

a. Infants and children are at high risk for elevated electrolyte levels from electrolyte replacement therapy

b. Feeding an infant improperly diluted infant formulas can cause renal damage from a hypertonic solute load

c. Feeding an infant cow's milk rather than formula or breast milk can cause hyperphosphatemia because of the higher P level in cow's milk

3. Older adults

a. Those taking diuretics or digitalis preparations are at particular risk for electrolyte imbalances, especially hypokalemia

b. Digitalis toxicity is a particular problem in this age-group because K, Ca, and Mg imbalances predispose to this condition

c. Inadequate water intake predisposes an older adult to excessive solute loads

d. Inadequate nutrition predisposes an older adult to electrolyte deficits, which may be aggravated by diuretic therapy

4. Chronically ill patients

a. Many chronic diseases—particularly renal failure, diabetes mellitus, and endocrine disorders—are considered etiologic factors in various electrolyte imbalances

b. Chronic illness impairs the body's ability to compensate for imbalances; monitor these patients closely

Points to Remember

Sodium imbalances are usually accompanied by fluid imbalances.

Potassium imbalances can lead to life-threatening cardiac dysfunction.

Calcium imbalances are associated with neuromuscular problems.

Infants and young children, older adults, and chronically ill patients are at increased risk for electrolyte imbalances.

Glossary

Chvostek's sign—physical assessment test for hypocalcemia involving lightly tapping the facial nerve (located on the upper cheek below the zygomatic bone); abnormal spasm of facial muscles points to hypocalcemia

Dysrhythmia—abnormal cardiac rhythm usually caused by alterations in normal cardiac conduction

Tetany—condition indicating abnormal calcium metabolism characterized by cramps, convulsions, muscle twitching, and sharp wrist and ankle joint flexion

Trousseau's sign—physical assessment test for hypocalcemia involving applying a blood pressure cuff to the upper arm and inflating it to a pressure 20 mm Hg above the patient's systolic blood pressure; carpal spasm points to hypocalcemia

Acid-Base Imbalances

Learning Objectives

After studying this section, the reader should be able to:

- List the four major types of acid-base imbalances.

- Describe the major alteration in carbon dioxide (CO_2) associated with respiratory acidosis and alkalosis.

- Describe the major alteration in bicarbonate (HCO_3) associated with metabolic acidosis and alkalosis.

- State the nursing implications for each acid-base imbalance.

VII. Acid-Base Imbalances

A. **Introduction**
   1. Acid-base imbalances are common clinical conditions that accompany any disorder
   2. The hydrogen (H) cation influences both electrolyte balance and acid-base balance
   3. Hydrogen ion concentration (pH) is measured through arterial blood gas (ABG) analysis
   4. Acid-base imbalances are categorized into four major types
      a. Respiratory acidosis
      b. Respiratory alkalosis
      c. Metabolic acidosis
      d. Metabolic alkalosis
   5. These major imbalances can occur in three forms
      a. Primary
      b. Mixed
      c. Compensated
   6. *Primary imbalances* originate from an acute condition such as respiratory acidosis resulting from hyperventilation syndrome
   7. *Mixed imbalances* involve both a metabolic and a respiratory imbalance occurring at the same time. Mixed imbalances occur when:
      a. One disturbance results in acidosis; the other, in alkalosis
      b. Both disturbances are acidosis
      c. Both disturbances are alkalosis
   8. *Compensated imbalances* involve the body's attempt to bring the pH back to normal after a primary imbalance has occurred; the body compensates for a primary imbalance by initiating the opposite imbalance. Compensated imbalances usually are associated with chronic disorders, such as chronic obstructive pulmonary disease (COPD)
   9. The body responds to an acid-base imbalance with a physiologic process known as *compensation*
      a. Respiratory imbalances are compensated for by the renal system
      b. Metabolic imbalances are compensated for by the respiratory system

B. **Respiratory acidosis**
   1. General information
      a. Respiratory acidosis is a primary acid-base imbalance resulting from altered alveolar ventilation leading to CO_2 retention
      b. Abnormally slow or shallow respirations or poor alveolar ventilation resulting in inadequate gas exchange causes CO_2 to accumulate in the lungs and the serum, increasing the levels of carbonic acid (H_2CO_3) circulating in the blood and lowering pH
      c. Low arterial pH and elevated serum CO_2 levels (hypercapnia) constitutes respiratory acidosis

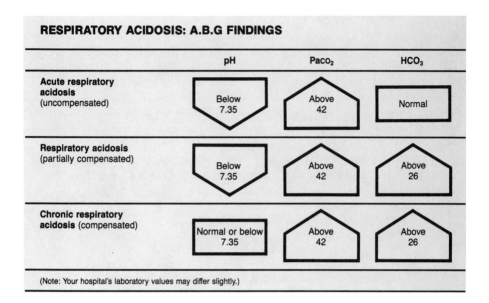

RESPIRATORY ACIDOSIS: A.B.G FINDINGS

	pH	Paco$_2$	HCO$_3$
Acute respiratory acidosis (uncompensated)	Below 7.35	Above 42	Normal
Respiratory acidosis (partially compensated)	Below 7.35	Above 42	Above 26
Chronic respiratory acidosis (compensated)	Normal or below 7.35	Above 42	Above 26

(Note: Your hospital's laboratory values may differ slightly.)

    d. Respiratory acidosis may be acute, as in sudden ventilatory failure, or chronic, as in emphysema

    e. The body attempts to compensate for respiratory acidosis by increasing renal reabsorption of HCO$_3$

2. Etiology
    a. Alveolar hypoventilation
    b. Acute abdominal distention (inhibits pulmonary excursion)
    c. Respiratory arrest
    d. Overdose of sedatives or anesthetic
    e. Airway obstruction
    f. COPD
    g. Congestive heart failure
    h. Pneumonia
    i. Cardiac arrest
    j. Pneumothorax or hydrothorax
    k. Chest wall injury, such as fractured ribs
    l. Amyotrophic lateral sclerosis
    m. Pulmonary fibrosis
    n. Pickwickian syndrome
    o. Cystic fibrosis
    p. Myasthenia gravis

3. Clinical manifestations
    a. Dyspnea
    b. Tachycardia

    c. Slow, shallow respirations
    d. Confusion
    e. Tremors
    f. Dizziness
    g. Convulsions
    h. Warm, flushed skin
    i. Asterixis
    j. Altered level of consciousness
    k. Cyanosis (a late sign)
4. Diagnostic findings (uncompensated)
    a. Arterial pH <7.35
    b. Partial pressure of CO_2 in arterial blood ($PaCO_2$) >42 mm Hg
    c. HCO_3 level 22 to 26 mEq/liter
5. Diagnostic findings (compensated)
    a. Arterial pH borderline (7.35 or lower)
    b. $PaCO_2$ > 42 mm Hg
    c. HCO_3 level > 26 mEq/liter
6. Nursing implications
    a. Encourage the patient to turn, cough, and deep-breathe every 2 hours, which improves ventilation; chest physiotherapy may also be ordered
    b. Maintain a patent airway through the use of such measures as suctioning to prevent CO_2 retention
    c. Monitor ABG levels for changes in pH and CO_2
    d. Monitor vital signs, particularly respiratory rate and depth, for changes that may indicate worsening acidosis
    e. Position the patient in the semi-Fowler's or orthopneic position to ease breathing
    f. Ensure that the patient drinks 2 to 3 liters of fluids per day (unless contraindicated), which will help liquefy secretions and aid their expulsion and promote adequate CO_2 exchange
    g. Administer supplemental oxygen, as ordered; do so cautiously in a patient with COPD, because excessive oxygen decreases or completely depresses the ventilatory drive and may worsen acidosis
    h. Monitor serum K levels for hyperkalemia because K moves out of the cell during respiratory acidosis
    i. Administer medications, as ordered, to treat the underlying respiratory dysfunction—for example, bronchodilators for bronchospasms, antibiotics for respiratory infection
    j. Administer sedatives cautiously; many sedatives depress the respiratory drive, which can lead to CO_2 accumulation
    k. Provide emotional support and reassurance to the patient, who likely will be quite anxious

C. Respiratory alkalosis
1. General information
   a. Respiratory alkalosis occurs when alveolar hyperventilation results in decreased serum CO_2 levels (hypocapnia), causing excessive CO_2 exhalation
   b. Decreased serum CO_2 levels lead to decreased H_2CO_3 production and, in turn, increased arterial pH
   c. Hyperventilation is the most common cause of respiratory alkalosis
   d. The body attempts to compensate for respiratory alkalosis by increasing renal excretion of HCO_3 (can take 24 to 48 hours)
2. Etiology
   a. Psychogenic conditions, such as hysteria or acute anxiety
   b. Hyperventilation syndrome
   c. Overventilation with mechanical ventilator
   d. Aspirin overdose
   e. Fever from septicemia
   f. Severe pain
   g. Central nervous system trauma or lesions
   h. Hypoxia
   i. Pregnancy
   j. Hyperventilation during labor and delivery
   k. Thyrotoxicosis
3. Clinical manifestations
   a. Rapid, deep respirations
   b. Light-headedness
   c. Headache
   d. Vertigo
   e. Decreased concentration and attention span
   f. Paresthesias
   g. Tetany
   h. Carpopedal spasm (Trousseau's sign)
   i. Tinnitus
   j. Palpitations
   k. Dry mouth
   l. Blurred vision
   m. Syncope
   n. Convulsions and coma
4. Diagnostic findings (uncompensated)
   a. $PaCO_2$ level <38 mm Hg
   b. Arterial pH >7.45
   c. Partial pressure of oxygen in arterial blood (PaO_2) normal or elevated (80 to 100)
   d. HCO_3 level 22 to 26 mEq/liter
5. Diagnostic findings (compensated)
   a. $PaCO_2$ level <38 mm Hg
   b. Arterial pH borderline (7.45 or slightly higher)

RESPIRATORY ALKALOSIS: A.B.G. FINDINGS

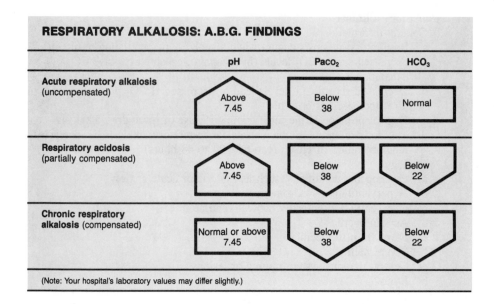

	pH	$Paco_2$	HCO_3
Acute respiratory alkalosis (uncompensated)	Above 7.45	Below 38	Normal
Respiratory acidosis (partially compensated)	Above 7.45	Below 38	Below 22
Chronic respiratory alkalosis (compensated)	Normal or above 7.45	Below 38	Below 22

(Note: Your hospital's laboratory values may differ slightly.)

    c. HCO_3 level <22 mEq/liter
    d. Serum potassium (K) level below 3.8 mEq/liter
    e. Urine pH alkaline (above 8)
    f. Serum calcium (Ca) level below 7 mg/dl
  6. Nursing implications
    a. Monitor vital signs, specifically respiratory rate and depth
    b. Instruct the patient to breathe slowly and less deeply to decrease CO_2 loss
    c. As necessary, have the patient breathe into a paper bag or use a rebreather mask to rebreathe CO_2
    d. Administer sedatives, as ordered, to slow the respiratory rate; monitor the patient carefully to guard against respiratory depression and CO_2 retention
    e. Intervene as necessary to correct the underlying cause of hyperventilation, such as pain or anxiety
    f. Monitor ABG values, particularly $PaCO_2$ levels, to evaluate the effectiveness of interventions
    g. If the patient is intubated, adjust mechanical ventilator settings to decrease ventilatory rate and depth
    h. Monitor serum K levels, especially in a patient with chronic hyperventilation, because K is exchanged for H ions and moves from the extracellular to the intracellular space, resulting in low serum levels
    i. Monitor laboratory results for values indicating compensation, such as decreased HCO_3 levels and normalization of pH; such values won't appear until at least 24 hours after onset of hyperventilation
    j. Provide emotional support and reassurance to help decrease anxiety

D. Metabolic acidosis
1. General information
   a. Metabolic acidosis results from excessive accumulation of fixed acids or loss of fixed bases in body fluids
   b. Fixed acids, such as hydrochloric acid (HCl), are produced by metabolism or ingested foods
   c. Chloride (Cl), a component of HCl, competes with HCO_3 for combination with sodium (Na); excessive Cl retention or ingestion increases fixed acid production. The kidneys' inability to retain sufficient HCO_3 to compensate results in an excess of H ions and, eventually, metabolic acidosis
   d. The major sign of metabolic acidosis is decreased arterial pH accompanied by decreased arterial HCO_3 levels
   e. Metabolic acidosis never results from a respiratory problem—with the exception of lactic acidosis from anaerobic metabolism (lack of available oxygen at the cellular level)
   f. Increased levels of circulating H ions result in rapid stimulation of peripheral chemoreceptors, which increases the respiratory rate within minutes of the onset of acidosis
   g. The body attempts to compensate for metabolic acidosis through hyperventilation, which results in decreased $PaCO_2$ levels; respiratory compensation begins within minutes but takes several hours to take full effect
2. Etiology
   a. Diabetic ketoacidosis
   b. Salicylate toxicity
   c. Acute or chronic renal failure
   d. Diuretic therapy resulting in excessive HCO_3 loss through the kidneys
   e. Total parenteral nutrition therapy
   f. Prolonged, severe diarrhea
   g. Fistula drainage (for example, pancreatic)
   h. Use of carbonic anhydrase inhibitors such as acetazolamide (Diamox)
   i. Alcohol intoxication
   j. Starvation
   k. Hypoxia
   l. Decreased tissue perfusion, as from trauma or burns
   m. High-fat diet
   n. Excessive gain of Cl, as from the administration of ammonium chloride
3. Clinical manifestations
   a. Kussmaul's respirations
   b. Lethargy
   c. Drowsiness
   d. Confusion
   e. Flushed, warm, dry skin
   f. Fruity breath
   g. Peripheral vasodilation

METABOLIC ACIDOSIS: A.B.G. FINDINGS

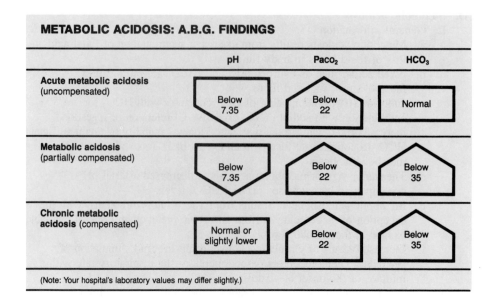

	pH	Paco$_2$	HCO$_3$
Acute metabolic acidosis (uncompensated)	Below 7.35	Below 22	Normal
Metabolic acidosis (partially compensated)	Below 7.35	Below 22	Below 35
Chronic metabolic acidosis (compensated)	Normal or slightly lower	Below 22	Below 35

(Note: Your hospital's laboratory values may differ slightly.)

      h. Nausea and vomiting
      i. Twitching
      j. Convulsions
      k. Stupor
      l. Coma
   4. Diagnostic findings (uncompensated)
      a. Arterial pH level <7.35
      b. Arterial HCO$_3$ level <22 mEq/liter
      c. PaCO$_2$ level 38 to 45 mm Hg
      d. Base excess negative
      e. Serum CO$_2$ level <18 mEq/liter
   5. Diagnostic findings (compensated)
      a. Arterial pH borderline (7.35 or slightly lower)
      b. Arterial HCO$_3$ level <22 mEq/liter
      c. PaCO$_2$ level <35 mm Hg
      d. Base excess negative
      e. Serum K level > 5.5 mEq/liter
      f. Urine pH ≤ 4.5
   6. Nursing implications
      a. Monitor patients at risk for metabolic acidosis, especially those with diabetes mellitus, sepsis, or shock
      b. Monitor vital signs, particularly respiratory rate and depth
      c. Monitor ABG values, particularly pH, because small decreases in pH indicate large increases in H ion concentration
      d. Monitor HCO$_3$ and K levels; low HCO$_3$ and high K levels may be an early indicator of acidosis

e. Administer sodium bicarbonate (NaHCO$_3$) cautiously through an existing I.V. line in a large vein
f. Institute cardiac monitoring for a patient with elevated serum K levels
g. As necessary, intervene to correct the underlying cause of acidosis; in many cases, correction of the underlying problem will resolve acidosis, precluding the need for more aggressive intervention, such as NaHCO$_3$ administration
h. Administer I.V. fluids containing lactate, unless contraindicated, as ordered; lactate is converted to HCO$_3$ in the liver
i. In a diabetic patient with metabolic acidosis linked to hyperglycemia, administer insulin and normal saline solution to correct hyperglycemia; remember, insulin administration also will lower serum K levels
j. Administer I.V. fluids and oxygen to correct lactic acidosis linked to overexertion by decreasing hypoxemia and triggering a conversion to aerobic metabolism
k. In renal failure, drug overdose, or poisoning, expect to assist with peritoneal dialysis or hemodialysis to correct pH
l. In a patient with chronic acidosis, provide a diet high in carbohydrates and low in fat, which will decrease metabolic waste products and thus ameliorate acidosis

E. Metabolic alkalosis
1. General information
   a. Metabolic alkalosis results from excessive accumulation of fixed bases or excessive loss of fixed acids in body fluids
   b. A major cause of metabolic alkalosis is loss of a fixed acid, such as HCL, from the stomach, either through nasogastric (NG) suctioning or excessive vomiting
   c. Loss of a fixed acid increases the pH
   d. As pH increases, H ion concentration decreases
   e. As H ion concentration decreases, more H$_2$CO$_3$ dissociates and HCO$_3$ concentration increases through renal reabsorption
   f. This results in increased renal excretion of H, Cl, and K
   g. Cl competes with HCO$_3$ for combination with Na; when Cl levels fall, HCO$_3$ levels rise in compensation to balance the Na
   h. The body attempts to compensate for metabolic alkalosis through hypoventilation
   i. Stimulation of chemoreceptors is decreased, slowing respiratory rate and conserving CO$_2$
2. Etiology
   a. Excessive administration or ingestion of HCO$_3$
   b. Excessive loss of H ions from NG suctioning or vomiting
   c. Prolonged diuretic therapy, particularly K-wasting diuretics
   d. NaHCO$_3$ administration during cardiopulmonary resuscitation
   e. Hypokalemia
   f. Cushing's syndrome

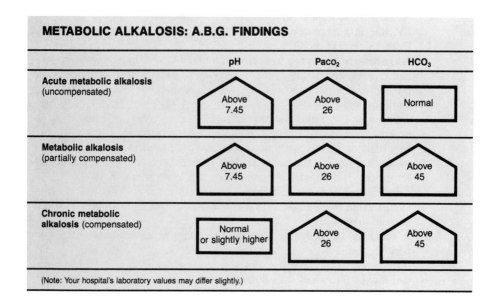

METABOLIC ALKALOSIS: A.B.G. FINDINGS

	pH	Paco$_2$	HCO$_3$
Acute metabolic alkalosis (uncompensated)	Above 7.45	Above 26	Normal
Metabolic alkalosis (partially compensated)	Above 7.45	Above 26	Above 45
Chronic metabolic alkalosis (compensated)	Normal or slightly higher	Above 26	Above 45

(Note: Your hospital's laboratory values may differ slightly.)

      g. Hyperaldosteronism
  3. Clinical manifestations
      a. Decreased respiratory rate and depth
      b. Dizziness
      c. Paresthesias in fingers and toes
      d. Circumoral paresthesias
      e. Carpopedal spasm
      f. Muscle hypertonicity
      g. Nausea and vomiting
      h. Confusion
      i. Irritability
      j. Agitation
      k. Convulsions
      l. Coma
  4. Diagnostic findings (uncompensated)
      a. Arterial pH >7.45
      b. Arterial HCO$_3$ level >26 mEq/liter
      c. PaCO$_2$ level 38 to 45 mm Hg
      d. Base excess positive
      e. Serum CO$_2$ level >28 mEq/liter
  5. Diagnostic findings (compensated)
      a. Arterial pH borderline (7.45 or slightly higher)
      b. Arterial HCO$_3$ levels >26 mEq/liter
      c. PaCO$_2$ level >45 mm Hg
      d. Base excess positive

    e. Serum K and Cl levels (relative to Na) decreased

6. Nursing implications

    a. Monitor patients at risk for metabolic alkalosis, particularly those with gastric fluid losses from long-term NG suctioning or vomiting

    b. Assess fluid intake and output to determine the amount of gastric fluid loss

    c. Monitor vital signs, especially respirations, which will usually decrease as the body attempts to conserve CO_2

    d. As necessary, intervene to correct the underlying cause of the imbalance; for example, control vomiting by administering an antiemetic

    e. Administer I.V. fluid and electrolyte supplements, as ordered, to replace fluid volume, K, and Cl losses; monitor electrolyte studies to prevent overreplacement

    f. Remember, sufficient Cl must be supplied to enable renal absorption of Na with Cl and subsequent renal excretion of excessive HCO_3

    g. Monitor heart rate and rhythm to detect hypokalemia; a 12-lead ECG may be indicated

    h. Warn the patient and family about the dangers of excessive HCO_3 ingestion; explain that alkalosis can develop from overuse of antacids or $NaHCO_3$

    i. Teach a patient taking a K-wasting diuretic to watch for and report symptoms of hypokalemia, such as weakness and excessive urine output; teach the patient and family how to replace K by either increased dietary intake or oral supplements

Points to Remember

Respiratory acidosis results from CO_2 retention.

Respiratory alkalosis most commonly results from hyperventilation.

Metabolic acidosis results from excessive accumulation of fixed acids or excessive loss of fixed bases.

Metabolic alkalosis results from excessive loss of fixed acids or excessive accumulation of fixed bases.

Glossary

Asterixis—hand-flapping tremor commonly accompanying metabolic disorders

Hyperventilation—rapid respiratory rate commonly associated with anxiety

Hypoventilation—abnormally reduced respiratory rate and depth

Thyrotoxicosis—life-threatening disorder associated with pronounced hyperthyroidism; also known as Graves' disease

Fluid and Electrolyte Replacement Therapy

Learning Objectives

After studying this section, the reader should be able to:

• List the administration routes for pure water.

• List two examples of isotonic and hypotonic crystalloid solutions.

• Compare and contrast colloids and blood products.

• Discuss the nursing implications associated with each route of fluid and electrolyte replacement therapy.

VIII. Fluid and Electrolyte Replacement Therapy

A. Introduction

1. Fluid and electrolyte replacement therapy is aimed at restoring and maintaining homeostasis
2. Goals of replacement therapy include
   a. Correcting fluid and electrolyte losses
   b. Meeting daily fluid and electrolyte needs
   c. Preventing new imbalances
   d. Preserving renal function
3. The type of fluid or electrolyte selected for replacement is determined after establishing the type of fluid or electrolyte imbalance
4. Methods of fluid and electrolyte replacement therapy include
   a. Oral and gastric feedings
   b. Parenteral therapy
5. Factors affecting choice of replacement therapy include
   a. Patient's overall health status
   b. Patient's renal status
   c. Patient's age
   d. Patient's usual maintenance requirements
   e. Type of imbalance
   f. Severity of imbalance
6. Administration routes
   a. Oral route: oral ingestion of fluids and electrolytes as liquids or solids administered directly into the GI tract
   b. Nasogastric (NG) route: instillation of fluids and electrolytes through feeding tubes, such as NG, gastrostomy, and jejunostomy tubes
   c. Intravenous (I.V.) route: administration of fluids and electrolytes directly into the bloodstream; this route may be accomplished by continuous infusion, bolus, or I.V. push injection
7. Replacement therapy fluids are categorized by their concentration (tonicity); they are usually prepared in isotonic, hypotonic, and hypertonic concentrations
8. *Isotonic* solutions have the same osmolality as plasma, approximately 310 mEq/liter
   a. Infusion of isotonic fluids does not alter vascular space osmolality
   b. Isotonic fluids expand the intracellular and extracellular spaces equally
   c. The degree of intracellular fluid (ICF) and extracellular fluid (ECF) expansion correlates with the amount of fluid infused
   d. Examples of isotonic solutions include dextrose 5% in water (D_5W), 0.9% sodium chloride, dextrose 5% and 0.9% sodium chloride, Ringer's solution, and lactated Ringer's solution
9. *Hypotonic* solutions have a lower osmolality than plasma, approximately 250 mEq/liter
   a. Infusion of hypotonic solutions may cause hypo-osmolality because these solutions have a lower concentration of electrolytes than does plasma

    b. Hypotonic fluids transcend all membranes from vascular space to tissue to cell

    c. Water intoxication is a serious potential complication of excessive hypotonic fluid administration

    d. Examples of hypotonic solutions include dextrose 5% and 0.45% sodium chloride, and dextrose 5% and 0.25% sodium chloride

10. *Hypertonic* solutions have a higher osmolality than plasma, usually >375 mEq/liter

    a. Infusion of hypertonic solutions can raise plasma osmolality significantly

    b. Hypertonic fluid administration can cause vascular volume expansion and ICF deficit

    c. Complications of excessive administration of hypertonic solutions include excessive vascular volume and potential for pulmonary edema and heart failure

    d. Examples of hypertonic solutions include whole blood, albumin, total parenteral nutrition, concentrated dextrose solution (10% and greater), fat emulsions, elemental oral diets, and tube feedings

11. Nursing implications for administering oral fluid and electrolyte replacement therapy

    a. Work with the doctor to calculate the patient's daily fluid requirements

    b. Calculate the patient's total body surface area using a standard chart, to accurately determine fluid needs

    c. To meet the patient's daily fluid needs, administer 1,500 ml of water for each square meter of body surface area

    d. Position the patient in semi- or high-Fowler's position to ensure safe ingestion of fluids and to avoid aspiration

    e. Check the temperature of oral fluids before administration, to prevent oral mucosa burns and to promote ingestion

    f. Prepare foods and fluids as necessary, such as mixing replacement fluid with table foods, and provide portions compatible with appetite

    g. Provide a relaxed, pleasant environment to enhance the patient's appetite and promote compliance with therapy

    h. Maintain accurate fluid intake and output records

    i. Obtain the patient's daily weight, and correlate any weight gain or loss with the 24-hour total on the fluid intake and output record

    j. Increase the amount of fluid replacement to 2,400 ml per square meter of body surface area for moderate fluid losses and to 3,000 ml/m² for severe fluid losses

    k. Assess the effectiveness of fluid replacement therapy by monitoring urine output, serum sodium levels, blood urea nitrogen levels, and serum osmolality

    (See Appendix D: *Standard I.V. Solutions Used for Fluid and Electrolyte Replacement*, pages 114-115)

12. Nursing implications for administering NG tube feedings

    a. Constitute tube feedings as ordered or use preconstituted liquid tube feedings to prevent administration of hypertonic fluids

  b. Position the patient in semi-Fowler's or upright to prevent aspiration

  c. Remember, intubated patients should have the endotracheal tube cuff deflated during feedings

  d. Before administering the feeding, check NG tube placement by injecting air into the tube and auscultating the stomach for a gurgling sound; this step is not necessary for gastric and jejunostomy tubes, which are surgically positioned

  e. Check for retention of formula by withdrawing aspirant; volume >160 ml indicates retention

  f. Make sure that feedings are at room temperature to prevent abdominal cramping on administration

  g. Wean the patient gradually onto hypertonic tube feeding. Start hypertonic feedings with small diluted amounts, approximately 50 to 60 ml per feeding, in an effort to prevent diarrhea. Isotonic tube feedings may be started at full strength

  h. Administer adequate amounts of water via the parenteral route when necessary to meet total fluid needs

  i. Consider using a mechanical feeding pump for continuous infusion to prevent possible fluid overload

  j. Use clean equipment and technique—especially for gastrostomy and jejunostomy tubes, which carry a high infection risk because the peritoneum is entered

13. Nursing implications for administering parenteral fluid and electrolyte replacement therapy

  a. Assess veins, degree of limb mobility, and type of fluid ordered for infusion to determine the optimal site for parenteral line placement

  b. Use appropriate equipment for each specific purpose—for example, a butterfly needle for temporary infusions and an intracatheter for long-term therapy or for infusion of irritating solutions or medications

  c. Label and time-tape the bottle or bag to ensure proper administration rate

  d. Apply a dressing at the insertion site after stabilizing the needle with tape to prevent infection; follow with an arm board to immobilize the arm

  e. Calculate and adjust the flow rate, as ordered, to prevent fluid overload

  f. Change dressings according to institutional protocol; assess the insertion site for redness, tenderness, and swelling

  g. Infuse hypertonic solution cautiously; rapid infusion could precipitate heart failure. Use of an infusion control pump is recommended

  h. Administer protein infusions after 3 to 4 days of carbohydrate infusion (the daily protein requirement for adults is 1 g/kg of body weight; for children, 1 to 2 g/kg)

  i. Assess the compatibility of all medications with the type of fluid being administered to prevent complications (for example, D_5W and dilantin are incompatible)

      j. Consider vitamin administration after 3 days of parenteral therapy to prevent possible vitamin deficiencies

B. Water
1. General information
   a. Most water is ingested orally and directly
   b. Water also can be ingested indirectly in fruits, vegetables, and meats
2. Uses: replacement of pure water losses
3. Administration routes
   a. Oral route
   b. NG route
4. Nursing implications (See Section VIII.A.11 on nursing implications for oral fluid and electrolyte replacement)

C. Crystalloids
1. General information
   a. Crystalloid solutions are used primarily for hydration and replacement therapy
   b. Crystalloid solutions are composed mainly of water with dissolved electrolytes or dextrose
   c. Crystalloid solutions can be isotonic, hypertonic, or hypotonic
   d. Isotonic crystalloids include D_5W, 0.9% sodium chloride, and lactated Ringer's solution
   e. Hypertonic crystalloids include dextrose 10% in water and dextrose 50% in water
   f. Hypotonic crystalloids include 0.45% sodium chloride and 0.25% sodium chloride
2. Composition
   a. Water
   b. Carbohydrates: solutions contain dextrose in 5% to 50% concentrations
   c. Electrolytes: solutions can include sodium (Na), chloride (Cl), and other electrolytes
   d. Acid-base components: acetate, lactate, or ammonium chloride
3. Types
   a. D_5W contains 50 g of dextrose and water
   b. 0.9% sodium chloride contains water, 154 mEq/liter of Na, and 154 mEq/liter of Cl
   c. Dextrose 5% and 0.45% sodium chloride contains water, dextrose, 77 mEq/liter of Na, and 77 mEq/liter Cl
   d. Dextrose 5% and 0.25% sodium chloride contains water, dextrose, 34 mEq/liter of Na, and 34 mEq/liter of Cl
   e. Ringer's solution contains water and a range of electrolytes, including 130 mEq/liter of Na, 109 mEq/liter of Cl, 4 mEq/liter of K, and 3 mEq/liter of Ca
   f. Lactated Ringer's solution contains water and all the electrolytes listed for Ringer's solution plus 28 mEq/liter of lactate

4. Uses
   a. Provide hydration
   b. Provide calories
   c. Spare protein from use as a source of energy (D_5W)
   d. Correct Na and Cl deficits (0.9% sodium chloride)
   e. Replace ECF losses (0.9% sodium chloride)
   f. Correct acidosis (lactated Ringer's solution)
5. Administration routes
   a. I.V. infusion
   b. I.V. bolus
6. Nursing implications
   a. Keep in mind that nursing implications are similar to those for parenteral replacement therapy (see Section VIII.A.12)
   b. Administer 0.9% sodium chloride to correct Na or Cl deficits

D. Nutritional supplements: Enteral
1. General information
   a. Nutritional supplements are administered to restore or maintain a patient's nutritional status
   b. These supplements contain essential nutrients, such as amino acids, calories, electrolytes, and vitamins
2. Composition
   a. Elemental diets: combination of water and a powdered mixture of essential and nonessential amino acids, fatty acids, glucose, electrolytes, and minerals
   b. Tube feedings: liquid mixture of water, protein, carbohydrates, fats, minerals, and vitamins; can be commercially prepared or liquefied whole foods
3. Types
   a. Hyperosmolar elemental diets, such as Vivonex
   b. Hyperosmolar tube feedings, such as Ensure and Sustacal
   c. Iso-osmolar tube feedings, such as Osmolite and Isocal
4. Uses
   a. Provide a caloric supplement
   b. Restore and maintain nutritional status
   c. Provide an additional energy source
5. Administration routes
   a. Oral route
   b. NG route
   c. Gastric route through gastrostomy or jejunostomy tube
6. Nursing implications: similar to those for oral and NG tube feedings (see Section VIII.A.11)

E. Nutritional supplements: Parenteral
1. General information
   a. Parenteral nutritional supplements are administered to restore or maintain a patient's nutritional status

    b. They contain essential nutrients, such as amino acids, caloric sources, electrolytes, and often vitamins

    c. Parenteral supplements are administered through a peripheral or central I.V. line

    d. Total parenteral nutrition (TPN) provides a concentrated source of calories (approximately 1,000 calories/liter) as well as total nutrient requirements; TPN is administered through a central I.V. line

    e. Approximately 400 calories/day must be administered to spare protein; a total of 1,600 calories per day is required to meet daily adult energy needs

    f. Protein requirements for adults average 1 g/kg of body weight; for children, 1 to 2 g/kg

    g. Ethyl alcohol provides a rich source of calories; 1 g of alcohol yields approximately 7 calories

    h. Alcohol solutions usually are administered with D_5W

2. Composition

    a. Carbohydrate parenteral nutrients: composed of carbohydrates available as dextrose solutions in concentrations of 5% to 50%

    b. Protein parenteral solutions: composed of crystalline amino acids or colloidal elements

    c. Fat emulsions: composed of lipids in 10% and 20% concentrations

    d. TPN: composed of dextrose (25% to 50%), amino acids, and selected amounts of K, Na, calcium, phosphorus, and magnesium. Water and fat-soluble vitamins also may be included

    e. Alcohol solutions: contain ethyl alcohol, a rich source of calories

    f. Vitamins: may include both fat soluble and water soluble

3. Types

    a. Crystalline amino acids or albumin-type products

    b. Fat emulsions

    c. Ethyl alcohol solutions

    d. Vitamin C, B-complex, or fat-soluble

4. Uses

    a. Provide calories

    b. Restore and maintain nutritional status

    c. Spare protein (if 400 calories/day are administered)

    d. Provide an additional energy source

5. Administration route: I.V. infusion

6. Nursing implications

    a. Keep in mind that nursing implications are similar to those for parenteral replacement therapy (see Section VIII.A.12)

    b. Be aware that fat emulsions are incompatible with electrolyte and most other solutions

    c. Do not use filters when administering fat emulsions

    d. Remember, fat emulsions are contraindicated in patients who cannot metabolize fats—for example, patients with pancreatitis

    e. Assess for adverse reactions—such as vomiting, headache, dyspnea, allergic reaction, hyperlipidemia, temperature elevation, flushing, sweating, hepatomegaly, and shock—when administering fat emulsions

    f. Use a mechanical infusion pump for TPN administration because the patient is at risk for hyperosmolality with rapid infusion

    g. Infuse TPN through a central line only

    h. Assess the patient every 15 minutes during the first hour of TPN therapy to determine tolerance, then every 30 minutes thereafter

    i. Consider using a 0.22-micron filter for TPN infusion; this size inhibits passage of *Pseudomonas* bacteria and decreases the risk of contamination

    j. Use meticulous sterile technique when changing TPN central line dressings; the patient is at high risk for infection because of the solution's concentrated glucose content

    k. Assess laboratory studies, such as serum BUN, creatinine, and electrolyte levels, every 12 to 24 hours (or whenever the patient's condition changes) for indications of an imbalance

    l. Be aware that the common imbalances associated with TPN infusion include hyperkalemia, azotemia, hypophosphatemia, and metabolic acidosis

    m. Monitor for signs and symptoms of hyperglycemia; consider the need for insulin if hyperglycemia occurs

F. Colloids
1. General information
   a. Colloids are administered during acute situations to expand intravascular volume and maintain blood pressure
   b. Colloids are indicated for patients with a protein deficit, as found in starvation, liver disease, or alcohol (ETOH) abuse
2. Composition
   a. Plasma: composed of water, protein, and small amounts of carbohydrates and lipids
   b. Serum protein and albumin: composed of albumin and globulins
3. Types
   a. Fresh frozen plasma
   b. Albumin (Albumisol)
   c. Plasma protein fraction (Plasmanate)
4. Uses
   a. Restore serum protein levels
   b. Restore albumin levels
   c. Expand intravascular volume
   d. Correct hypotensive episodes
5. Administration routes
   a. I.V. infusion
   b. I.V. bolus

6. Nursing implications
   a. Keep in mind that nursing implications are similar to those for parenteral replacement therapy (see Section VIII.A.12)
   b. Be aware that colloid administration can greatly expand intravascular volume, putting the patient at risk for congestive heart failure
   c. Assess the patient's response to colloid administration by monitoring blood pressure, pulse, and central venous pressure readings
   d. Monitor serum protein and albumin levels for deficits during colloid administration

G. Blood and blood products
1. General information
   a. Normal adult blood volume averages about 75 ml/kg of body weight
   b. A plasma volume deficit of 15% to 20% is associated with hypovolemic shock
2. Types
   a. Whole blood
   b. Packed red blood cells
   c. Plasma
   d. Platelets
   e. Cryoprecipitate
3. Composition
   a. Blood: volume of 500 ml containing erythrocytes and all coagulation factors except VIII and V, but lacking platelets
   b. Packed red blood cells: volume of 250 to 300 ml containing erythrocytes and 100 ml plasma
   c. Plasma: plasma volume of 200 to 250 ml containing all coagulation factors but lacking platelets (a colloid)
   d. Platelets: plasma volume of 50 ml containing platelets
   e. Cryoprecipitate: plasma volume of 10 to 25 ml containing Factor VIII and fibrinogen
4. Uses
   a. Replace blood loss
   b. Replace red blood cell (RBC) loss
   c. Treat anemia
   d. Expand blood volume
5. Administration routes: I.V. infusion
6. Nursing implications
   a. Use principles of infection control when handling blood and blood products
   b. Use a blood filter when administering blood or blood products
   c. Inspect the blood bag's contents for discoloration
   d. Before administration, check blood identification information against patient information, following institutional protocol
   e. Assess blood temperature before administering, and use blood-warming

equipment when necessary

f. Take and record baseline vital signs before blood administration, including temperature, pulse, blood pressure, and respirations

g. Adjust infusion rate to avoid the danger of bacterial growth and RBC hemolysis from infusion hanging too long; the maximum infusion time is 4 hours

h. Monitor the patient's response to blood or blood product infusion throughout the first 15 minutes of infusion, then every 20 to 30 minutes

i. Assess for signs and symptoms of blood transfusion reaction, such as fever, chills, shortness of breath, headache, and hematuria

j. Monitor for signs and symptoms of anaphylactic reaction, including respiratory distress, hypotension, rash, flushing, chills, and pruritus

k. Watch for possible complications of massive transfusion, such as hyperkalemia, acidosis, hypothermia, citrate toxicity, and 2,3-diphosphoglycerate deficiency
   (See Appendix E: *Blood Component Therapy,* pages 116-117)

Points to Remember

Replacement fluids are available in three concentrations: isotonic, hypotonic, and hypertonic.

Colloids are used to expand vascular volume.

Too-rapid administration of hypertonic I.V. fluids can cause rapid vascular volume expansion and intracellular fluid deficit, leading to pulmonary edema.

Significant blood loss is replaced with blood products.

Glossary

Colloid—solution composed of serum proteins and albumin in plasma

Crystalloid—solution composed of water and solutes (primarily electrolytes) administered for hydration

Gastrostomy—surgically created opening into the stomach through the abdominal wall for insertion of a feeding tube

Parenteral fluid—solution administered intravenously

Conditions Associated with Fluid, Electrolyte, and Acid-Base Imbalances

Learning Objectives

After studying this section, the reader should be able to:

• Identify common conditions associated with fluid, electrolyte, and acid-base imbalances.

• Describe the specific imbalances involved in each of these conditions.

• Discuss how the pathophysiology of these conditions leads to imbalances.

• Discuss specific nursing implications for the imbalances occurring with each condition.

IX. Conditions Associated with Fluid, Electrolyte, and Acid-Base Imbalances

A. **Introduction**
1. Various conditions—particularly those affecting major regulatory systems—commonly result in fluid, electrolyte, or acid-base imbalances
2. Various conditions can disrupt the regulatory mechanism or action of an organ or system
3. Treatment instituted to correct a condition also can cause imbalances
4. Conditions involving excessive gains or losses of fluid, as occurs in diuretic therapy, nasogastric suctioning, vomiting, or diarrhea, or after massive tissue destruction (as in burns and trauma), will result in fluid, electrolyte, and acid-base imbalances
5. Imbalances commonly result from:
   a. Dietary restrictions
   b. Electrolyte replacement therapy
   c. Hormonal therapy (steroids)

B. **Renal failure**
1. General information
   a. The renal system is a major regulator of fluid, electrolyte, and acid-base balance
   b. Renal failure involves disruption of normal kidney function; it is classified as acute renal failure (ARF) or chronic renal failure (CRF)
   c. Both ARF and CRF affect the kidneys' functional unit, the nephron
   d. ARF occurs suddenly and is usually reversible; CRF occurs slowly and insidiously and is irreversible
   e. Imbalances occur as the kidneys lose the ability to excrete water, electrolytes, wastes, and acid-base products via the urine
   f. Patients with renal failure are at risk for fluid volume, electrolyte, and metabolic acid-base imbalances
   g. Other problems caused by renal failure that alter homeostasis include anemia, hypertension, uremia, and osteodystrophy
2. Pathophysiology
   a. The kidneys do not receive adequate blood flow because of diminished renal perfusion, either partial or complete bilateral obstruction, or nephron damage
   b. As a result, the kidneys cannot produce normal amounts of urine
   c. With abnormal urine production, the kidneys' ability to maintain homeostasis is altered
3. Potential imbalance: Extracellular fluid (ECF) volume excess
   a. Water and sodium (Na) retention during renal failure are associated with oliguria or anuria when the body cannot to excrete excess fluid
   b. This state can result in hypertension, peripheral edema, or pulmonary edema

4. Potential imbalance: ECF volume deficit
   a. Water losses in renal failure are associated with a diuretic or polyuric phase of ARF
   b. Dehydration occurs during the diuretic phase only when the large volume of urine output is not matched by adequate fluid replacement
   c. This state can result in hypotension and circulatory collapse
5. Potential imbalance: Hyperkalemia
   a. Hyperkalemia usually occurs with oliguria because potassium (K) excretion is reduced as urine output is diminished
   b. In CRF, the patient tends to tolerate high K levels; symptoms may not appear until the K level exceeds 7.5 mEq/liter
   c. In ARF, symptoms appear much earlier, often with K levels of 6 mEq/liter
6. Potential imbalance: Hypocalcemia
   a. The patient with hypocalcemia is at high risk for tetany and seizures; secondary hyperparathyroidism occurs after repeated episodes of significant hypocalcemia has caused the parathyroid gland to hypertrophy
   b. The overactive, enlarged parathyroid gland mobilizes calcium from bone to replenish the hypocalcemic serum
   c. Bone softening—known as osteomalacia or renal rickets—occurs in the patient with repeated episodes of hypocalcemia
7. Potential imbalance: Hyperphosphatemia
   a. Hyperphosphatemia results because the kidneys lose the ability to excrete phosphate
   b. It typically occurs in chronic renal failure when the glomerular filtration rate drops below 25 to 30 ml/minute
8. Potential imbalance: Hypermagnesemia
   a. Hypermagnesemia usually occurs secondary to abuse of magnesium-containing agents, such as laxatives (MOM) and antacids
   b. Hypermagnesemia should be suspected if the patient demonstrates sudden changes in neurologic status
9. Potential imbalance: Hypernatremia (less common) resulting from excessive Na and water retention
10. Potential imbalance: Metabolic acidosis
    a. Metabolic acidosis occurs commonly in ARF and CRF
    b. It develops as the kidneys lose the ability to secrete hydrogen ions (an acid) in the urine
11. Potential imbalance: Metabolic alkalosis
    a. Metabolic alkalosis rarely occurs in renal failure
    b. It usually occurs only after excessive administration of bicarbonate in an effort to correct metabolic acidosis
12. Nursing implications
    a. Assess the patient carefully to determine the type and extent of fluid, electrolyte, or acid-base imbalance
    b. Maintain an accurate fluid intake and output record; remember to calculate insensible water losses to determine fluid balance

     c. Obtain daily weight and correlate results with the 24-hour intake and output record

     d. Monitor vital signs, including lung sounds and central venous pressure when available, to detect fluid abnormalities; report hypertension that may occur secondary to fluid and Na retention

     e. Observe for signs and symptoms of fluid overload, such as edema, bounding pulse, and shortness of breath

     f. Monitor serum electrolyte levels for abnormalities

     g. Observe for signs and symptoms that may indicate electrolyte imbalance, such as tetany, paresthesias, and muscle weakness

     h. Monitor ECG readings to detect changes secondary to hypokalemia, hyperkalemia, hypocalcemia, hypercalcemia, hypomagnesemia, and hypermagnesemia

     i. As necessary, restrict electrolyte intake, especially K and P, to prevent further imbalances

     j. Monitor arterial blood gas (ABG) studies for pH; observe for symptomatic acidosis

     k. Administer diuretics, as ordered, to patients whose kidneys can still respond to remove fluid excess (glomerular filtration rate should be at least 25 ml)

     l. Administer such medications as oral electrolyte replacements and cation exchange resins as ordered, to correct electrolyte imbalances (see Section VI for specific interventions)

     m. Expect to administer sodium bicarbonate intravenously to control acute acidosis and orally to control chronic acidosis

     n. Be aware of the high Na content in a dose of sodium bicarbonate (approximately 50 mEq in one 50-ml ampule). Multiple doses may result in significant hypernatremia, which could contribute to the onset of heart failure and pulmonary edema

     o. Teach the patient and family how to calculate and record amounts (in milliliters) of fluid ingested and excreted

     p. Teach the patient and family about electrolyte content in solid foods, fluids, and medications—especially over-the-counter antacids and laxatives—to prevent ingestion of excessive electrolytes

     q. Be prepared to initiate dialysis for electrolyte and acid-base imbalances that do not respond to medication therapy, or when fluid removal is not possible

     r. Determine the optimal "dry weight" for the dialysis patient. Dry weight is individualized for each patient and obtained after dialysis

C. Congestive heart failure (CHF)
  1. General information

     a. In CHF, the heart cannot pump sufficient blood volume to meet the body's metabolic demands

    b. CHF may result from conditions within or affecting the heart itself (such as cardiomyopathy, atherosclerotic heart disease, or acute myocardial infarction), from inadequate venous return (as in chronic obstructive pulmonary disease and pulmonary hypertension), from circulatory overload (as in excessive vascular volume expansion), or from albumin or mannitol infusion

    c. In left-sided CHF, the left ventricle cannot propel the blood volume forward into the aorta; blood backs up in the pulmonary vascular bed, increasing pulmonary capillary pressure and resulting in pulmonary venous congestion

    d. In right-sided CHF, the right ventricle has difficulty propelling the blood forward into the pulmonary circulation; blood backs up into the systemic circulation, causing blood pooling in the liver and increased pressure in the peripheral circulation, resulting in edema

    e. Patients with CHF are at risk for fluid volume, electrolyte, and metabolic acid-base imbalances

    f. Imbalances may result from the heart's failure to pump and to adequately perfuse the tissues, from stimulation of the renin-angiotensin-aldosterone mechanism, or from treatment interventions, such as diuretics

2. Pathophysiology

    a. The failing heart cannot generate the energy necessary to propel the ventricular blood volume forward

    b. Blood backs up in the system

    c. Cardiac output and hydrostatic pressure in the vascular space fall, which is reflected in a drop in blood pressure

    d. The kidneys, sensitive to the renal hypoperfusion state resulting from decreased cardiac output, trigger the renin-angiotensin-aldosterone mechanism

    e. Angiotensin II, produced from the conversion of renin and angiotensin I, acts directly on the vessels to produce a massive peripheral vasoconstriction and also stimulates the release of aldosterone, which enhances Na reabsorption at the nephron level

    f. Cardiac muscle pumping against a vasoconstricted vessel results in an increased work load (increased afterload) and exacerbates failure

    g. The Na reabsorption is accompanied by water reabsorption; these mechanisms cause an increased vascular volume, which compounds the existing cardiac compromise

3. Potential imbalance: ECF volume excess

    a. ECF volume excess is the most common fluid imbalance associated with CHF

    b. It results from the heart's failure to propel blood forward and consequent vascular pooling, and from the Na and water reabsorption triggered by the renin mechanism

    c. ECF volume excess commonly causes peripheral edema

4. Potential imbalance: ECF volume deficit usually associated with overaggressive diuretic therapy

5. Potential imbalance: Hypokalemia caused by prolonged diuretic use without adequate K replacement
6. Potential imbalance: Hyponatremia
   a. Hyponatremia may result from sodium loss due to diuretic abuse
   b. In some cases, it may result from a dilutional effect caused by greater water reabsorption than Na reabsorption
7. Potential imbalance: Hypernatremia
   a. Hypernatremia may occur if diuretic use produces much greater water loss than Na loss
   b. It also may be linked to an overactive renin mechanism causing excessive Na reabsorption
8. Potential imbalance: Hypochloremia resulting from excessive diuretic therapy
9. Potential imbalance: Metabolic acidosis
   a. Metabolic acidosis is linked to excessive lactic acid production.
   b. The lactic acid buildup results from significantly reduced tissue perfusion in a compromised individual
10. Potential imbalance: Metabolic alkalosis caused by excessive diuretic use leading to secretion of hydrochloric acid (HCl)
11. Nursing implications
    a. Monitor Na and water intake, as ordered, because hyponatremia and fluid volume deficit can stimulate the renin-angiotensin-aldosterone mechanism and exacerbate CHF. Usually, a mild Na restriction—such as no added salt—with no water restriction is implemented
    b. Monitor fluid status; check daily weight and fluid intake and output for significant changes
    c. Monitor vital signs, including blood pressure, pulse, respirations, and lung sounds for abnormalities that might indicate a fluid excess or deficit
    d. Assess for signs and symptoms of impending cardiac failure, such as fatigue; restlessness; rapid, thready pulse; hypotension; rapid respirations; dyspnea; coughing; decreased urine output; and liver enlargement
    e. Assess for the presence, amount, and location of edema; note the presence and degree of any pitting
    f. Monitor serum electrolyte levels, such as Na and K, for changes that may indicate an imbalance
    g. Administer such medications as digoxin, diuretics, and K supplements, as ordered, to support cardiac function and minimize symptoms
    h. Administer oral K supplements in orange juice or with meals to promote absorption and prevent gastric irritation

D. Respiratory insufficiency
1. General information
   a. The lungs are a major regulator of fluid, electrolyte, and acid-base balance
   b. In respiratory insufficiency, the lungs cannot maintain adequate gas exchange

    c. Respiratory insufficiency may result from hypoxemia secondary to increased pulmonary capillary pressure or permeability (for example, in left-sided CHF or pneumonia); from conditions impairing normal carbon dioxide (CO_2) elimination (such as chronic obstructive pulmonary disease or asthmatic crisis); or from neuromuscular impairment of respiratory drive, as can occur in drug overdoses, spinal cord injury, multiple sclerosis, or myasthenia gravis

    d. Patients with respiratory insufficiency are at risk for fluid volume, electrolyte, and respiratory acid-base imbalances

    e. Imbalances result from ventilatory impairment, which leads to excessive CO_2 retention or elimination or to excessive fluid losses through the lungs

2. Pathophysiology

    a. Inadequate oxygenation results in hypoxemia, leading to hypocapnia and an increased respiratory rate

    b. An increased respiratory rate leads to increased insensible fluid loss through the lungs and excessive elimination of CO_2

    c. Insufficient respiratory center stimulation results in hypercapnia, leading to hypoxemia

    d. Airway obstruction results in CO_2 retention and hypercapnia limiting the amount of CO_2 eliminated by the lungs; respiratory rate may be normal or increased

3. Potential imbalance: Respiratory acidosis

    a. Respiratory acidosis results from the lungs' inability to eliminate adequate amounts of CO_2

    b. Excessive CO_2 combines with water (H_2O) to form carbonic acid (H_2CO_3)

    c. Increased H_2CO_3 levels result in decreased pH, contributing to respiratory acidosis

4. Potential imbalance: Respiratory alkalosis

    a. Respiratory alkalosis results from too-rapid respirations, causing excessive CO_2 elimination

    b. The loss of CO_2 decreases the serum's acid-forming potential, resulting in respiratory alkalosis

5. Potential imbalance: ECF volume excess

    a. Prolonged respiratory treatment, such as nebulizers, can lead to the inhalation of water vapor and its absorption through lung tissue; excessive fluid absorption may also result from increased pulmonary capillary pressure or permeability

    b. This excessive fluid absorption can precipitate pulmonary edema

6. Potential imbalance: ECF volume deficit

    a. Water as vapor normally is eliminated during respiration

    b. Excessive water loss occurs in fever or any condition that increases the metabolic rate and thus the respiratory rate

7. Nursing implications

    a. Monitor ABG levels to assess oxygenation and pH status

      b. Assess lung status; monitor rate, depth, and character of respirations, making sure to check lung sounds for abnormalities

      c. Administer oxygen, as ordered, to help maintain adequate oxygenation and restore the normal respiratory rate

      d. Administer oxygen to the patient with COPD cautiously, because adequate serum oxygen levels depress the stimulus for breathing

      e. Perform chest physiotherapy and postural drainage as needed to promote adequate ventilation

      f. As necessary, intervene to correct the underlying respiratory problem and respiratory-based alterations in acid-base status

      g. Monitor fluid status by maintaining accurate fluid intake and output records

      h. Evaluate serum electrolyte levels for abnormalities that can occur with acid-base imbalances

E. Burns
  1. General information
      a. A burn refers to the destruction of the epidermis, dermis, or subcutaneous layers of the skin that can result from radiation; mechanical injury, such as friction; chemicals; electrical injury, such as lightning or electrical wires; or thermal injury, such as fire or frostbite

      b. Imbalances associated with burns result from alterations in skin integrity and internal body membranes and from the effect of heat on body water and solute losses that result from cellular destruction

      c. The type and severity of the imbalance depend on the burn type and depth, the percentage of body surface area involved, and the burn phase

      d. The percentage of body surface area involved is determined by the "rule of nines"; the greater the body surface involved, the greater the potential for imbalances

      e. Burn depth is classified as first-, second-, or third-degree

      f. *First-degree burns* (superficial partial thickness) involve superficial injury to the epidermis marked by an uncomplicated erythematous area; because the skin barrier remains intact, fluid loss is not a problem

      g. *Second-degree burns* (dermal partial thickness) involve damage to the epidermis, progressing to the dermis; blisters are present, and capillary damage is possible. Regeneration of the epithelial layer may occur

      h. *Third-degree burns* (full thickness) involve all skin layers; regeneration is not possible. Skin appearance is altered significantly and elasticity is lost. Skin color varies from red to black to white

      i. Third-degree burns carry the greatest risk of imbalances

      j. Burn phases refers to the stages that describe physiologic changes that occur after a burn. They include the fluid accumulation phase, fluid remobilization phase, and the convalescent phase

  2. Pathophysiology
      a. About 10% of plasma volume is lost into the tissue early after a severe burn because of edema caused by increased capillary permeability

    b. Further extravasation into areas other than the tissue, such as cells and third spaces, accounts for losses sometimes greater than 40%. Evaporation of water secondary to the heat loss from skin destruction results in an even greater volume loss, accounting for as much as 4 liters/day

    c. Intravascular water is rich in serum proteins, electrolytes, and essential minerals. Damaged capillaries at the burn site leak their fluid into the interstitial space, resulting in solute deficits

    d. Decreased tissue perfusion precipitates lactic acid formation

    e. Diminished respiratory excursion may cause CO_2 retention

    f. Disruption of the natural skin barrier promotes fluid losses and also increases the risk of infection

3. Potential imbalance: ECF volume deficit

    a. In burns, ECF volume deficit involves both extravasated fluid and fluid losses

    b. Composition of fluid losses resembles intravascular fluid that contains proteins and serum electrolytes

    c. Blood loss also may occur, adding to fluid volume losses

4. Potential imbalance: ECF volume excess

    a. ECF volume excess usually develops 3 to 5 days after a major burn injury

    b. It occurs as fluid shifts from the interstitial space back to plasma

5. Potential imbalance: Hyperkalemia

    a. In burns, hyperkalemia results from massive cellular trauma, metabolic acidosis, or renal failure

    b. It develops as K is released into the ECF during the fluid accumulation phase

6. Potential imbalance: Hyponatremia

    a. Hyponatremia results from increased intracellular water and Na losses

    b. Large amounts of Na are trapped in edema fluid and burn exudate

    c. Na is also lost when diuresis occurs during the fluid remobilization phase

7. Potential imbalance: Hypocalcemia

    a. Hypocalcemia can develop in burns as Ca travels to the damaged tissue and becomes immobilized at the burn site

    b. Hypocalcemia may occur 12 to 24 hours after the burn

8. Potential imbalance: Hypokalemia

    a. In burns, hypokalemia develops as K shifts from the ECF into the cells

    b. Hypokalemia usually occurs 4 to 5 days after a major burn injury

9. Potential imbalance: Metabolic acidosis

    a. Tissue perfusion becomes ineffective because of intravascular fluid shifts and overall fluid losses

    b. Fixed acids released from injured tissues accumulate, causing a drop in pH

10. Potential imbalance: Respiratory acidosis secondary to inadequate ventilation

11. Nursing implications

    a. Administer I.V. fluid therapy, as ordered, to restore depleted vascular volume; lactated Ringer's solution is usually the solution of choice

b. Calculate the amount of fluid replacement necessary; infuse 50% of this volume in the first 8 hours postburn and the remainder over the next 16 hours, as ordered

c. Do not adminster colloid solutions in the immediate postburn period; colloids will increase osmotic pressure in the interstitial space, which may exacerbate burn edema and increase the risk of vascular collapse

d. Remember, maintenance I.V. fluid replacement is based on daily assessment of fluid, electrolyte, acid-base, and nutritional needs

e. Administer I.V. electrolyte replacement therapy, as ordered, during the initial postburn period; monitor for signs and symptoms of hypokalemia, hyponatremia, and hypocalcemia

f. Use the oral route for electrolyte replacement as soon as the patient can tolerate it; patients usually experience a paralytic ileus after burns

g. Assess for signs and symptoms of metabolic acidosis and possibly respiratory acidosis secondary to impaired ventilation

h. Provide oxygen therapy, as ordered, to promote optimal respiratory function; consider mechanical ventilation for a patient with inadequate ventilation for any reason, especially smoke inhalation

i. Promote respiratory airway excursion to ensure adequate gas exchange

j. Maintain blood pressure within the normal range to ensure adequate tissue perfusion and to prevent lactic acid production

k. Assess for upper airway obstruction secondary to smoke inhalation; monitor for signs and symptoms, such as tachypnea, hoarseness, wheezing, and stridor

l. Assess skin for location, depth, and extent of burn

m. Assess cardiac and hemodynamic status for changes that indicate fluid imbalance

n. Monitor ECG readings for changes pointing to fluid and electrolyte imbalances, especially K imbalances

o. Assess fluid and hydration status, including skin turgor, daily weight, and hourly urine output for significant changes

p. Monitor ABG values and serum electrolyte levels to detect any significant changes

q. Assess the patient's nutritional status; total parenteral nutrition (TPN) may be necessary to meet the patient's increased metabolic needs

r. Perform burn care as ordered; monitor the patient's response

s. Observe the patient for signs and symptoms of infection, such as fever, tachycardia, and purulent wound drainage because the patient has an increased risk of infection exacerbated by destruction of the skin barrier and nutrient losses

F. Diabetic ketoacidosis (DKA)
1. General information
   a. DKA is an acute condition resulting from insulin deficiency in a patient with insulin-dependent diabetes

    b. In DKA, insufficient insulin is available to metabolize glucose; this may result from the patient's failure to take the prescribed insulin dose or from additional stressors, such as infection, trauma, or surgery

    c. DKA is characterized by hyperglycemia, ketonuria, hyperosmolality, ketonemia, and acidosis

    d. Imbalances occur primarily as a result of hyperglycemia

2. Pathophysiology

    a. Insufficient insulin results in an inability to metabolize glucose, as reflected by elevated serum glucose levels (exceeding 200 mg/dl)

    b. Fats are then burned for energy, resulting in ketosis (ketones are metabolic body acids)

    c. Large volumes of glucose in the serum create elevated serum osmolality

    d. Elevated glucose levels in the renal tubules precipitate osmotic diuresis with losses of water, Na, Cl, and K

    e. Significant dehydration and electrolyte deficits follow inadequate volume replacement

    f. These deficits trigger pulmonary and renal compensatory mechanisms

    g. The lungs attempt to eliminate excess acids through deep and rapid respirations (Kussmaul respirations) to compensate for the increase in metabolic acids (ketones)

    h. The kidneys attempt to increase acid excretion in the urine (ketonuria)

3. Potential imbalance: ECF volume deficit

    a. ECF volume deficit results from osmotic diuresis

    b. Excessive water is lost as the kidneys attempt to rid the body of excess acids

4. Potential imbalance: Hypokalemia

    a. Hypokalemia in DKA results from osmotic diuresis

    b. ECF volume deficit increases aldosterone secretion, which in turn leads to K loss

    c. Intracellular movement of K in response to ketone accumulation can exacerbate the imbalance

5. Potential imbalance: Hyponatremia secondary to osmotic diuresis

6. Potential imbalance: Hypophosphatemia secondary to treatment for DKA

7. Potential imbalance: Metabolic acidosis

    a. In DKA, fats are broken down for energy into ketones

    b. Ketones (strong acids) accumulate in the blood, increasing the amount of fixed acids and thus lowering the pH

8. Nursing implications

    a. Carefully monitor serum glucose and electrolyte levels, serum osmolality, and ABG results

    b. Monitor daily weight and intake and output records; insert an indwelling (Foley) catheter in a comatose patient to monitor urine output accurately

    c. Administer insulin, as ordered, correlating dosage with serum glucose levels

    d. Provide initial rehydration with 0.9% sodium chloride or lactated Ringer's solution, as ordered; rapid volume replacement may necessitate a rate as rapid as 1 liter/hour

e. Be prepared to administer bicarbonate for severe acidosis that does not respond to insulin

f. Assess hemodynamic parameters to determine the amount of volume replacement necessary to maintain adequate blood pressure and urine output

g. Avoid creating a hypoglycemic state with fluid replacement therapy; a rapid change in serum osmolality can precipitate cerebral edema

h. Replace K gradually with I.V. fluids; correction of metabolic acidosis releases K from cells

G. Hyperglycemic hyperosmolar nonketotic coma (HHNC)

1. General information

a. HHNC is an acute condition characterized by insulin deficiency in a patient with diabetes

b. In HHNC, some insulin is present but not enough to metabolize glucose

c. HHNC is characterized by hyperglycemia, hyperosmolality, and osmotic diuresis; ketosis and ketonuria do not occur

COMPARING DKA AND HHNC

Parameter	DKA Usually occurs in known Type I diabetic patients	HHNC Usually occurs in Type II diabetic patients (condition may be undiagnosed)
Precipitating factors	Undiagnosed diabetes, neglected treatment, injection, cardiovascular disorders, physical stress, emotional distress	Undiagnosed diabetes, infection or other stress, acute or chronic illnesses, certain ddrugs and medical procedures, severe burns treated with high sugar concentrations
Symptom onset	Slow (hours to days)	Slow (hours to days), but less gradual than DKA
Signs and symptoms Skin and mucous membranes	Warm, flushed, dry, loose skin; dry, crusty muscous membranes; soft eyeballs	Warm, flushed, dry, extremely loose skin; dry, crusty mucous membranes; soft eyeballs
Neurologic status	*Initial*—dullness, confusion, lethargy; diminished relfexes *Late*—coma	*Initial*—dullness, confusion, lethargy, diminished reflexes *Late*—coma
Muscle strength	Extremely weak	Extremely weak
Gastrointestinal	Anorexia, nausea, vomiting, diarrhea, abdominal tenderness and pain	None
Temperature	Possible fever (from dehydration or infection)	Possible fever (from dehydration)
Pulse	Mild tachycardia, weak	Usually rapid
Blood pressure	Subnormal	Subnormal

(continued)

COMPARING DKA AND HHNC *(continued)*

Respirations	*Initial*—deep, fast *Late*—Kussmaul's	Rapid (but no Kussmaul's)
Breath odor	Fruity, acetone	Normal
Weight	Decreased	Decreased
Other	Thirst	Thirst
Laboratory findings Blood glucose level	Above normal	Markedly above normal
Serum sodium level	Normal or subnormal	Above normal, normal
Serum potassium level	(Normal or above normal initially) subnormal	(Normal or above normal initially) subnormal
Serum ketones	Positive/large	Negative/small
Serum osmolarity	Above normal but usually less than 330 mOsm/liter	Markedly above normal— 350 to 450 mOsm/liter
Hematocrit	Above normal	Above normal
Arterial blood gasses	Metabolic acidosis with compensatory respiratory alkalosis	Normal
Urine glucose level	Above normal	Markedly above normal
Urine ketones	Positive/large	Negative/small
Urine output	*Initial*—polyuria *Late*—oliguria	Markedly above normal
Treatment	Insulin, fluid replacement, electrolyte replacement, antiacidosis therapy (if needed)	Fluid replacement, insulin, electrolyte replacement

    d. HHNC typically occurs in middle-aged or elderly patients with the onset of diabetes; it also may develop as a severe exacerbation of previously non-insulin-dependent diabetes

    e. Imbalances associated with HHNC include fluid volume and electrolyte imbalances that result primarily from osmotic diuresis

  2. Pathophysiology

    a. Insulin is present in sufficient amounts to prevent ketosis but in insufficient amounts to prevent hyperglycemia

    b. Hyperglycemia results in hyperosmolality and osmotic diuresis

    c. The urine contains relatively greater amounts of water than Na

  3. Potential imbalance: ECF volume deficit related to osmotic diuresis

  4. Potential imbalance: Hypernatremia resulting from proportionately greater water loss than Na loss

  5. Potential imbalance: Hypokalemia resulting from osmotic diuresis

  6. Potential imbalance: Hypophosphatemia secondary to osmotic diuresis

  7. Nursing implications

    a. Administer hypotonic 0.9% sodium chloride, as ordered; if volume

deficit is severe, use 0.9% sodium chloride to expand plasma volume at the prescribed flow rate to prevent overload
  b. Assess hydration status by monitoring intake and output, daily weight, and skin turgor for changes indicating imbalances
  c. Monitor serum glucose and electrolyte levels and plasma osmolality for changes
  d. Administer insulin, as ordered, adjusting insulin dosage to serum glucose levels
  e. Evaluate renal function before administering K replacement; K can be added to the I.V. fluid or given as an oral supplement
  f. Be aware that severe hypophosphatemia may be treated with potassium phosphate (K_2PO_4); carefully monitor patients receiving K_2PO_4 for hyperphosphatemia, especially a patient with diminished renal function

H. Syndrome of inappropriate antidiuretic hormone (SIADH)
  1. General information
    a. SIADH is characterized by inappropriate secretion of antidiuretic hormone (ADH)
    b. SIADH may result from head trauma, central nervous system disorders, pulmonary disorders, endocrine disorders, and use of certain medications, such as osmotic diuretics
    c. Imbalances associated with SIADH include fluid volume and electrolyte imbalances
  2. Pathophysiology
    a. Secretion of ADH is continuous and inappropriate
    b. Prolonged ADH secretion results in water retention, which leads to serum hypoosmality
    c. Urine osmolality is greater than serum osmolality
    d. Water reabsorption in the tubules increases, resulting in increased intravascular fluid volume
    e. The glomerular filtration rate increases, inhibiting the reabsorption of Na and water
    f. Increased intravascular fluid volume inhibits the release of renin and aldosterone, resulting in further urine Na losses
  3. Potential imbalance: ECF volume excess
    a. Tubular reabsorption of water is increased because of continued ADH secretion
    b. Water is retained, leading to increased intravascular fluid volume
  4. Potential imbalance: Hyponatremia
    a. Hyponatremia occurs as a result of aldosterone inhibition
    b. Decreased aldosterone secretion results in further urine Na losses
  5. Nursing implications
    a. Maintain accurate intake and output records; monitor for fluid intake exceeding output
    b. Monitor daily weight for increases; correlate weights with fluid gains or losses; remember, 1 liter of fluid weighs approximately 2¼ lb

    c. Monitor serum Na levels for abnormalities, and assess for signs and symptoms of hyponatremia; monitor serum and urine osmolality for changes

    d. In severe SIADH, expect to administer I.V. hypertonic saline solution to replace Na; when doing so, use a volume control device to prevent overload

    e. Expect to administer a diuretic—usually furosemide— concomitantly with I.V. hypertonic saline solution to promote water excretion

    f. Restrict daily fluid intake to approximately 500 to 700 ml, depending on urine output; remember to consider all intake routes when imposing fluid restrictions

    g. Intervene as appropriate to treat the underlying cause of SIADH

    h. Institute safety precautions to minimize risk of injury in patients with changes in sensorium

I. Postoperative response

1. General information

    a. The preoperative and operative phases are major stressors triggering the physiologic stress response, which may affect fluid, electrolyte, and acid-base balance

    b. The symptoms associated with the postoperative phase imbalances result from the body's stress response

    c. Resolution of this phase is marked by a diuretic phase

    d. Studying the postoperative response provides a perspective on how the body responds to other stressors

    e. Imbalances resulting from surgery include fluid volume, electrolyte, and metabolic acid-base imbalances

    f. Surgery can cause deficiencies of all electrolytes; these deficiencies may persist if not corrected

2. Pathophysiology

    a. The sympathetic response causes increased heart rate and contractility, and vasoconstriction

    b. Adrenocorticotropic hormone stimulates the release of mineralocorticoids and glucocorticoids

    c. The mineralocorticoids, primarily in the form of aldosterone, stimulate the reabsorption of Na and water at the renal tubules

    d. The glucocorticoids promote the mobilization of fats and the breakdown of protein and glycogen; glucocorticoids also suppress the immune system, increasing the patient's susceptibility to infection

    e. The stress response stimulates the hypothalamus. which leads to ADH release

    f. The adrenal medulla is stimulated to release increased amounts of norepinephrine and epinephrine, leading to intense vasoconstriction

    g. Systemic vasoconstriction causes localized reduction in renal blood flow, triggering the renin-angiotensin-aldosterone mechanism and leading to further vasoconstriction and Na and water retention

3. Potential imbalance: ECF volume excess
   a. In most cases of ECF volume excess, ADH, aldosterone, and renin combine to promote excessive reabsorption of Na and water
   b. ECF volume excess also may result from overadministration of Na-containing fluids in the first few postoperative days
4. Potential imbalance: ECF volume deficit resulting from internal or external fluid loss associated with surgical procedure or fluid status before the procedure
5. Potential imbalance: Third-space shifting
   a. Third-space shifting results from surgery's effect on tissue injury
   b. A third space is created around the operative site
   c. Fluids move to this third space and edema forms in and about the operative site during the first few postoperative days.
6. Potential imbalance: Hyponatremia
   a. Hyponatremia is common in the first or second postoperative day
   b. It commonly results from excessive ADH secretion in response to stress
   c. It also may be caused by excessive administration of I.V. fluids such as dextrose 5% in water (D_5W)
7. Potential imbalance: Hypokalemia
   a. Hypokelmia can result from increased K excretion due to increased secretion of mineralocorticoids and glucocorticoids
   b. K losses secondary to a surgical procedure also contribute to hypokalemia
8. Potential imbalance: Respiratory acidosis
   a. Respiratory acidosis commonly results from diminished ventilation and respiratory depression due to anesthesia or narcotics
   b. It also may result from impaired oxygen exchange, as in atelectasis or airway obstruction
   c. It also may be linked to decreased respiratory depth due to abdominal distention or postoperative pain
9. Potential imbalance: Metabolic acidosis
   a. Postoperative metabolic acidosis usually is secondary to the surgical tissue destruction resulting in increased hydrogen (H) ion production
   b. Reduced urine output also reduces H ion secretion
   c. Metabolic acidosis also can result from excessive losses of intestinal, bile, or pancreatic juices
10. Potential imbalance: Metabolic alkalosis
    a. Postoperative metabolic alkalosis commonly occurs in patients who have lost a large amount of gastric secretions
    b. It is closely associated with hypokalemia and hypochloremia
11. Nursing implications
    a. Anticipate the possibility of postoperative phase imbalances resulting from the physiologic aspects of the patient's stress response
    b. Promote stress reduction: Provide preoperative teaching, allow family visits, keep the patient informed about recovery progress, and encourage expression of feelings and concerns

    c. Provide adequate nutrition (calories, protein, vitamins, minerals) to counteract the catabolic effect of glucocorticoids, to replace nutrients, to promote healing, and to prevent infection

    d. Assess patient progress by monitoring vital signs, intake and output, and daily weight

    e. Assess wound drain sites for amount and character of drainage and record

    f. Support the patient's return to a homeostatic state by promoting regular ambulation, turning, coughing, and deep breathing

    g. Administer I.V. fluid replacement therapy as ordered

    h. Monitor serum electrolyte levels for abnormalities

J. Intestinal obstruction

1. General information
   a. Intestinal obstruction involves interference with the normal peristaltic movement of intestinal contents
   b. Obstruction may result from a physical barrier or from impairment of bowel innervation resulting in an inability to move the digested food forward
   c. Imbalances associated with intestinal obstruction include fluid volume and metabolic acid-base imbalances

2. Pathophysiology
   a. A bowel obstruction causes hyperperistalsis and trauma to the intestinal wall
   b. Intestinal gas and fluid accumulate proximal to the obstruction
   c. Large quantities of water and electrolytes are secreted into the bowel and form a third space
   d. Plasma proteins enter the intestinal lumen, causing increased distention
   e. The portion of the intestines above the obstruction continues to secrete more fluid; the edematous bowel cannot absorb this large fluid volume, leading to increased distention and volume depletion

3. Potential imbalance: ECF volume deficit resulting from trapped fluid in the intestines, prolonged vomiting, or excessive GI suctioning; volume loss may be 5 liters or more

4. Potential imbalance: Third-space shifting
   a. The altered bowel wall contributes to the formation of an abnormal compartment
   b. Third-space shifting results from fluid accumulation in this abnormal space

5. Potential imbalance: Metabolic acidosis
   a. Metabolic acidosis may result from vomiting larger amounts of alkaline intestinal fluids than acidic gastric fluids
   b. The vomiting usually occurs from obstruction in the distal small intestines

6. Potential imbalance: Metabolic alkalosis (rare) resulting from excessive vomiting of large amounts of gastric fluid

7. Potential imbalance: Respiratory acidosis, usually linked to marked abdominal distention, which increases pressure on the diaphragm and impairs respiratory excursion
8. Nursing implications
   a. Administer I.V. isotonic or hypotonic solutions (usually lactated Ringer's solution or D$_5$W) to replace fluid losses; administer at the prescribed rate to prevent overload
   b. Remember, isotonic 0.9% sodium chloride may be used if gastric fluid loss is excessive
   c. Administer Na and K replacements based on the patient's serum electrolyte levels; monitor these levels closely to prevent imbalances
   d. Assess hydration status by monitoring intake and output, daily weight, and skin turgor
   e. Monitor vital signs, especially pulse rate and blood pressure, to detect changes indicating fluid imbalance
   f. Evaluate the need for TPN or alternate feeding methods to maintain or restore nutritional status
   g. Assess the presence and character of bowel sounds and stool quantity and character to detect resolution of obstruction
   h. Monitor GI suction for amount and character of drainage
   i. Prepare the patient for possible surgical intervention

K. Excessive GI fluid loss
1. General information
   a. GI fluid loss may include loss of saliva, gastric juices, bile, pancreatic juice, and intestinal secretions
   b. All GI fluids are isotonic—except saliva, which is hypotonic
   c. GI fluid loss is the most common cause of fluid and electrolyte imbalances
   d. GI fluids may be lost through excessive vomiting, gastric suctioning, diarrhea, intestinal suctioning, ileostomy, and fistulas
2. Pathophysiology
   a. Gastric, intestinal, and pancreatic fluids contain large amounts of Na, K, and Cl
   b. Gastric fluid is highly acidic; intestinal and pancreatic fluids and bile are alkaline
   c. Loss of gastric fluids through vomiting or gastric suctioning results in loss of acid, specifically HCl
   d. Loss of intestinal and pancreatic juices and bile through diarrhea, intestinal suctioning, fistulas, and ileostomy results in loss of alkaline fluids
   e. Losses of either type result in loss of Na, K, and Cl
3. Potential imbalance: ECF volume deficit
   a. ECF volume deficit can result from both gastric and intestinal fluid losses
   b. Large amounts of fluid, including water, can be lost if the condition causing the loss is prolonged and not corrected

4. Potential imbalance: Metabolic alkalosis
    a. Metabolic alkalosis can result from prolonged vomiting or gastric suctioning
    b. H and Cl in gastric fluid are lost in large amounts
5. Potential imbalance: Metabolic acidosis
    a. Metabolic acidosis can result from prolonged diarrhea, intestinal suctioning, or excessive ileostomy drainage
    b. Bicarbonate ions in intestinal fluids are lost in large quantities
6. Potential imbalance: Hypokalemia from prolonged loss of gastric or intestinal fluid
7. Potential imbalance: Hyponatremia from prolonged vomiting, diarrhea, or gastric or intestinal suctioning
8. Nursing implications
    a. Measure and record the amount of fluid lost by vomiting, suctioning, or diarrhea
    b. Assess hydration status, including intake and output, daily weight, and skin turgor; remember to include GI losses as part of output
    c. Administer oral fluids containing water and electrolytes (such as Gatorade and Pedialyte) if the patient can tolerate fluids; maintain the patient on nothing-by-mouth (NPO) status if he cannot tolerate fluids
    d. Administer I.V. fluids, as ordered, for replacement; monitor the infusion rate and volume to prevent overload
    e. Check tube placement often if the patient has gastric suctioning to prevent possible fluid aspiration
    f. Irrigate the suction tube with isotonic 0.9% sodium chloride, as ordered; remember, plain water is never used for irrigation because it may potentiate fluid and electrolyte imbalances
    g. Restrict the amount of ice chips given to the patient; too much water from ice chips can cause further electrolyte imbalances
    h. Administer such medications as antiemetics or antidiarrheals, as ordered, to control the underlying problem
    i. Evaluate serum electrolyte levels to detect further abnormalities and to monitor the effectiveness of therapy

Points to Remember

Renal dysfunction often leads to the retention of fluids, electrolytes, acid-base components, and wastes.

In CHF, imbalances may result from the heart's failure to pump and to adequately perfuse the tissues, from stimulation of the renin-angiotensin-aldosterone mechanism, or from treatment interventions, such as diuretics.

Imbalances linked to respiratory insufficiency result from ventilatory impairment leading to excessive CO_2 retention or elimination or fluid losses through the lungs.

Fluid loss in burns results from evaporation, heat loss, and ECF losses secondary to increased vascular permeability.

Endocrine problems, such as DKA, HHNC, and SIADH, lead to numerous imbalances resulting from altered hormonal regulation.

Postoperative response is a physiologic stress response that affects the body's fluid, electrolyte, and acid-base balance.

Fluid loss from the GI tract can be alkaline (intestinal) or acidic (gastric).

Glossary

Glucocorticoid—steroid secreted from the adrenal cortex that is involved with the postoperative stress response

Mineralocorticoid—substance secreted from the adrenal cortex, such as aldosterone, that causes Na retention in renal tubules

Renin-angiotensin-aldosterone mechanism—renal mechanism that increases blood pressure by causing peripheral vasoconstriction and Na and water retention

Sympathetic response—reaction by a part of the autonomic nervous system that increases the heart rate and causes peripheral vasoconstriction

Appendices

Appendix A

FLUID BALANCE CHECKLIST

Below is a quick reference checklist to assess a patient's fluid balance status. Remember your priorities are to establish baseline vital signs and weight, then to monitor and record daily vital signs, weight, and fluid intake and output.

ASSESSMENT CHECKLIST	PROBLEMS
Monitor weight	
☐ Loss of 5% or less ☐ Loss of 5% to 10% ☐ Loss of more than 10%	Mild dehydration Moderate dehydration Severe dehydration
☐ Gain of 5% or less ☐ Gain of 5% to 10% ☐ Gain of more than 10%	Mild overhydration Moderate overhydration Severe overhydration
Observe eyes	
☐ Dry conjunctiva ☐ Decreased tearing ☐ Periorbital edema ☐ Sunken eyes ☐ Soft eyeballs	Fluid volume deficit
Observe mouth	
☐ Sticky, dry mucous membranes	Fluid volume deficit Sodium excess
☐ Increased viscosity of saliva	Sodium deficit
Observe lips	
☐ Dry, cracked	Fluid volume deficit
Observe tongue	
☐ Longitudinal furrows	Sodium deficit
Assess cardiovascular system	
☐ Increased pulse rate ☐ Decreased pulse rate ☐ Decreased blood pressure ☐ Narrow pulse pressure	Fluid volume deficit
☐ Bounding pulse ☐ Jugular vein distension	Fluid volume excess
☐ Cardiac dysrhythmias	Potassium deficit Magnesium deficit

FLUID BALANCE CHECKLIST *(continued)*

ASSESSMENT CHECKLIST	PROBLEMS
Assess respiratory system	
☐ Moist crackles, rhonchi ☐ Increased respiratory rate ☐ Dyspnea ☐ Pulmonary edema	Fluid volume excess
☐ Shallow, slow breathing	Respiratory alkalosis with or without metabolic acidosis
☐ Deep, rapid breathing	Respiratory acidosis with or without metabolic alkalosis
Assess GI system	
☐ Absent bowel sounds (ileus)	Potassium deficit
☐ Abdominal cramps	Potassium excess
☐ Nausea, vomiting, and diarrhea	Magnesium excess
☐ Nausea, diarrhea	Potassium excess
Assess renal system	
☐ Oliguria	Sodium deficit or excess Potassium excess
Observe extremities	
☐ Edema of dependent body parts (including sacrum and lower extremities)	Fluid volume excess
Observe skin condition	
☐ Warm	Sodium excess
☐ Cold ☐ Poor skin turgor	Fluid volume deficit
☐ Warm, moist	Fluid volume excess
☐ Flushing	Magnesium deficit
Assess neurologic condition	
☐ Depressed central nervous system	Fluid volume deficit Electrolyte imbalance
☐ Increased intracranial pressure	Sodium deficit
☐ Positive Babinski's sign	Magneisum deficit
☐ Disorientation or confusion	Fluid volume excess Acidosis or aklalosis Electrolyte imbalance
☐ Seizures	Calcium deficit Magnesium deficit

(continued)

FLUID BALANCE CHECKLIST *(continued)*

ASSESSMENT CHECKLIST	PROBLEMS
Observe musculoskeletal system	
☐ Muscle weakness	Potassium deficit Calcium excess
☐ Paralysis of flaccid muscles	Potassium excess
☐ Numbness in extremities	Potassium excess
☐ Hypertonicity (physical checks include positive Chvostek's sign, carpopedal spasm, Trousseau's sign)	Metabolic alkalosis Calcium excess Magnesium deficit
☐ Muscle rigidity	Metabolic alkalosis
Monitor laboratory test results	
☐ Hematocrit elevation	Fluid volume excess or deficit Sodium excess
☐ Protein elevation	None
☐ Protein depletion	Malnutrition Starvation Third-space shifting
☐ Increased urine pH	Metabolic and respiratory alkalosis
☐ Decreased urine pH	Metabolic and respiratory acidosis
☐ Elevated BUN and normal serum creatinine	Fluid volume deficit
Monitor urine specific gravity	
☐ Elevation	Fluid volume deficit
☐ Decrease	Sodium deficit
☐ Red blood cell increase	Sodium excess or deficit Fluid volume overload

Appendix B

SELECTED LABORATORY TESTS

The doctor may order any of the tests below to assess a patient's fluid and electrolyte status. (*Note:* Your hospital's laboratory may use slightly different values for the normal ranges shown here.)

SERUM TESTS

Serum sodium
Normal values: 135 to 145 mEq/liter
Implications of abnormal findings:
● Above normal—hypernatremia
● Below normal—hyponatremia

Serum potassium
Normal values: 3.5 to 5 mEq/liter
Implications of abnormal findings:
● Above normal—hyperkalemia
● Below normal—hypokalemia

Serum chloride
Normal values: 95 to 105 mEq/liter
Implications of abnormal findings:
● Above normal—hyperchloremia (possibly associated with excessive normal saline solution or ammonium chloride administration)
● Below normal—hypochloremia (commonly associated with hypokalemia and metabolic alkalosis)

Serum calcium
Normal values:
● Total serum calcium—8.5 to 10.5 mg/dl (4.0 to 5.5 mEq/liter)
● Serum ionized calcium—approximately 50% of total serum calcium level
Implications of abnormal findings:
● Above normal—acidosis
● Below normal—alkalosis
Note: Total serum calcium refers to the sum of serum ionized calcium and serum protein-bound calcium. Evaluate the patient's total serum calcium level in light of the serum albumin level—for every gram/deciliter that the serum albumin level falls or rises beyond normal, the serum calcium level falls or rises approximately 0.8 mg/dl.

Serum phosphate (phosphorus)
Normal values: 2.5 to 4.8 mg/dl (1.8 to 2.6 mEq/liter)
Implications of abnormal findings:
● Above normal—hyperphosphatemia
● Below normal—hypophosphatemia

Serum magnesium
Normal values: 1.5 to 2.5 mEq/liter (1.8 to 3.0 mg/dl)
Implications of abnormal findings:
● Above normal—hypermagnesemia
● Below normal—hypomagnesemia

Serum glucose
Normal values: 70 to 100 mg/dl
Implications of abnormal findings:
● Above normal—osmotic diuresis and hypovolemia
● Below normal—no clinically significant implications

Carbon dioxide (CO_2) content
Normal values: 24 to 30 mEq/liter
Implications of abnormal findings:
● Above normal—metabolic alkalosis (except in patients with chronic obstructive pulmonary disease)
● Below normal—metabolic acidosis (However, if the arterial pH value indicates alkalosis, below-normal CO_2 content signifies respiratory alkalosis.)
Note: CO_2 content reflects total serum bicarbonate and carbonic acid levels.

Serum osmolality
Normal values: 280 to 295 mOsm/kg
Implications of abnormal findings:
● Above normal—hypernatremia, hyperglycemia (may also accompany blood urea nitrogen elevation)
● Below normal—hyponatremia
Note: Serum osmolality depends mainly on the serum sodium level.

Serum proteins
Normal values:
● Serum total protein—6.0 to 8.0 g/dl
● Serum albumin—3.5 to 5.5 g/dl
● Serum globulin—1.5 to 3.0 g/dl
Implications of abnormal findings:
● Above normal—hypovolemia
● Below normal—intravascular–to–interstitial fluid shift (edema)
Note: Evaluate the serum albumin level in light of the patient's serum calcium level.

Blood urea nitrogen (BUN)
Normal values: 10 to 20 mg/dl
Implications of abnormal findings:
● Above normal—hypovolemia, excessive protein intake, increased catabolism
● Below normal—overhydration, reduced protein intake

Serum creatinine
Normal values: 0.7 to 1.5 mg/dl
Implications of abnormal findings:
● Above normal—severe hypovolemia, renal disease
● Below normal—no clinically significant implications

BUN:creatinine ratio
Normal values: 10:1
Implications of abnormal findings:
● Above normal (ratio increased in favor of BUN)—hypovolemia, low kidney perfusion pressure, increased protein metabolism
● Below normal (ratio decreased in favor of creatinine)—low protein intake, hepatic insufficiency (may also accompany repeated dialysis)
Note: When both BUN and creatinine levels increase but the 10:1 ratio remains, suspect intrinsic renal disease, or, in some cases, hypovolemia.

Hematocrit
Normal values:
● Men—44% to 52%
● Women—39% to 47%
Implications of abnormal findings:
● Above normal—hypovolemia
● Below normal—hypervolemia

URINE TESTS

Urine sodium
Normal values: 30 to 280 mEq/24 hours
Implications of abnormal findings:
● Above normal—increased salt intake, diabetic ketoacidosis, dehydration
● Below normal—decreased salt intake, acute renal failure, congestive heart failure

(continued)

SELECTED LABORATORY TESTS *(continued)*

Urine chloride
Normal values: 110 to 250 mEq/24 hours
Implications of abnormal findings:
• Above normal—dehydration, diabetic ketoacidosis
• Below normal—excessive diaphoresis, congestive heart failure, hypochloremic metabolic alkalosis
Note: A below-normal value may accompany prolonged vomiting or gastric suctioning.

Urine potassium
Normal values: 25 to 125 mEq/24 hours
Implications of abnormal findings:
• Above normal—dehydration
• Below normal—hypokalemia

Urine calcium
Normal values (may vary with dietary calcium intake):
• Men—less than 275 mg/24 hours
• Women—less than 250 mg/24 hours
Implications of abnormal findings:
• Above normal—hyperparathyroidism, vitamin D toxicity, renal tubular acidosis
• Below normal—hypoparathyroidism, renal insufficiency, vitamin D deficiency, thiazide diuretic use

Urine phosphate (phosphorus)
Normal values: Below 1,000 mg/24 hours

Implications of abnormal findings:
• Above normal—hyperparathyroidism, renal tubular acidosis
• Below normal—vitamin D toxicity, hypoparathyroidism, renal insufficiency

Urine magnesium
Normal values: Below 150 mg/24 hours
Implications of abnormal findings:
• Above normal—chronic renal disease, chronic alcoholism, adrenocortical insufficiency
• Below normal—acute or chronic diarrhea, diabetic ketoacidosis, dehydration, advanced renal failure, decreased dietary magnesium intake, or increased dietary calcium intake

Urine osmolality
Laboratory test: measures number of particles per unit of water in urine
Normal value: 50 to 1,200 mOsm/liter (depends on the circulating titer of antidiuretic hormone and the rate of urinary solute excretion)
Significance:
• Reflects changes in urine contents more accurately than specific gravity, depending on the previous state of hydration; urine osmolality should be 1½ times that of serum osmolality.

Urine specific gravity
Laboratory test: is inversely proportional to volume and measures urine concentration
Normal value: 1.010 to 1.030
Significance:
• Increases with any condition causing hypoperfusion of kidneys, leading to oliguria (for example, shock or severe dehydration)
• Decreases when tubules are unable to reabsorb water and concentrate urine

Urine pH
Laboratory test: measures the acidity or alkalinity of urine
Normal value: 4.5 to 8.0
Significance:
• Increases in metabolic and respiratory alkalosis, with magnesium ammonium phosphate stones or with certain urea-splitting infections (such as those caused by *Pseudomonas, Proteus,* and *Escherichia coli*)
• Decreases with uric acid stones and with metabolic and respiratory acidosis
• In renal acidosis, pH may be normal or slightly more acidic only when the plasma bicarbonate level is very low

Appendix C

ARTERIAL BLOOD GAS FINDINGS AND INTERPRETATIONS

To help determine a patient's acid-base status, use the chart below. Keep in mind that your hospital's laboratory may use values that differ slightly from those shown here.

pH	Paco₂	HCO₃⁻	IMPLICATION	CAUSE
Below 7.35	Normal	Below 22	Metabolic acidosis—uncompensated	Acid gain or base loss (causing base deficit)
Below 7.35	Below 35	Below 22	Metabolic acidosis—partially compensated	Acid gain or base loss (causing base deficit)
Normal	Below 35	Below 22	Metabolic acidosis—compensated	Acid gain or base loss (causing base deficit)
Below 7.35	Above 45	Normal	Respiratory acidosis—uncompensated	Hypoventilation
Below 7.35	Above 45	Above 26	Respiratory acidosis—partially compensated	Hypoventilation
Normal	Above 45	Above 26	Respiratory acidosis—compensated	Hypoventilation
Above 7.45	Normal	Above 26	Metabolic alkalosis—uncompensated	Base gain or acid loss (causing base excess)
Above 7.45	Above 45	Above 26	Metabolic alkalosis—partially compensated	Base gain or acid loss (causing base excess)
Normal	Above 45	Above 26	Metabolic alkalosis—compensated	Base gain or acid loss (causing base excess)
Above 7.45	Below 35	Normal	Respiratory alkalosis—uncompensated	Hyperventilation
Above 7.45	Below 35	Below 22	Respiratory alkalosis—partially compensated	Hyperventilation
Normal	Below 35	Below 22	Respiratory alkalosis—compensated	Hyperventilation
Below 7.35	Above 45	Below 22	Combined respiratory acidosis and metabolic acidosis	Hypoventilation, plus acid gain or base loss
Above 7.45	Below 35	Above 26	Combined respiratory alkalosis and metabolic alkalosis	Hyperventilation, plus base gain or acid loss
Variable (depends on which disorder is more severe)	Above 45	Above 26	Mixed respiratory acidosis and metabolic alkalosis	Hypoventilation, plus base gain or acid loss
Variable (depends on which disorder is more severe)	Below 35	Below 22	Mixed respiratory alkalosis and metabolic acidosis	Hyperventilation, plus acid gain or base loss

Appendix D

STANDARD I.V. SOLUTIONS USED FOR FLUID AND ELECTROLYTE REPLACEMENT

PRODUCT	OSMOLARITY	ELECTROLYTES	
		ELEMENT	AMOUNT
Dextrose solutions			
• 2.5%	126 mOsm/liter	N/A	N/A
• 5%	252 mOsm/liter	N/A	N/A
• 10%	505 mOsm/liter	N/A	N/A
• 20%	1,010 mOsm/liter	N/A	N/A
• 50%	2,525 mOsm/liter	N/A	N/A
Saline solutions			
• 0.45%	154 mOsm/liter	Sodium chloride	77 mEq/liter
• 0.9%	308 mOsm/liter	Sodium chloride	154 mEq/liter
• 3%	1,026 mOsm/liter	Sodium chloride	513 mEq/liter
• 5%	1,710 mOsm/liter	Sodium chloride	855 mEq/liter
Dextrose-saline solutions			
• 5% D/0.45 normal saline	406 mOsm/liter	Sodium chloride	77 mEq/liter
• 5% D/0.9 normal saline	559 mOsm/liter	Sodium chloride	154 mEq/liter
Ringer's (plain) solution	309 mOsm/liter	Sodium	147 mEq/liter
		Potassium	4 mEq/liter
		Calcium	4.5 mEq/liter
		Chloride	155.5 mEq/liter
Lactated Ringer's solution	273 mOsm/liter	Sodium	130 mEq/liter
		Potassium	4 mEq/liter
		Calcium	3 mEq/liter
		Chloride	109 mEq/liter
		Lactate	28 mEq/liter
Dextrose			
In lactated Ringer's solution			
• 2.5%	265 mOsm/liter	(see "Lactated	(see "Lactated
• 5%	525 mOsm/liter	Ringer's solution"	Ringer's solution"
• 10%	775 mOsm/liter	above)	above)
In Ringer's (plain) solution			
• 2.5%	N/A	(see "Ringer's [plain]	(see "Ringer's [plain]
• 5%	562 mOsm/liter	solution" above)	solution" above)
• 10%	N/A		
Dextran 40 and 70			
Dextran 40			
• 10% injection with 5% dextrose	252 mOsm/liter	Sodium	77 mEq/500 ml
• 10% injection with normal saline solution	308 mOsm/liter	Chloride	77 mEq/500 ml
Dextran 70			
• 6% injection with 5% dextrose	N/A	N/A	N/A
• 6% injection with normal saline solution	N/A	N/A	N/A
Mannitol			
• 5% in 0.45 normal saline	275 mOsm/liter	Sodium	77 mEq/liter
• 10% in 0.45 normal saline	550 mOms/liter	Chloride	
• 20% in 0.45 normal saline	1100 mOsm/liter	77 mEq/liter	

CALORIES/LITER AND INDICATIONS	PRECAUTIONS AND NURSING IMPLICATIONS
80 to 1,700 calories. Maintains water balance and correct imbalance. Supplies calories as carbohydrates.	Electrolyte-free solutions may cause peripheral circulatory collapse and anuria in patients with sodium deficiency. May aggravate hypokalemia and irritate veins. Do not administer with blood. Electrolyte-free solution increases body fluid loss.
No calories. Fluid replacement, dehydration, sodium depletion. Low-salt syndrome (hyponatremia).	Use chloride solution with caution in edematous patients with heart, renal, or hepatic disease. Administer slowly.
170 calories. Fluid replacement, caloric feeding, dehydration, sodium depletion.	Use chloride solution with caution in patients with compromised cardiovascular or pulmonary status. Continually assess for crackles, edema, and skin turgor.
No calories. Dehydration, sodium depletion, replacement of GI loss.	Assess laboratory values for correction of electrolyte imbalance. Continually assess for signs and symptoms of electrolyte imbalances.
9 calories. Replacement of surgical and GI loss, dehydration, sodium depletion, acidosis, diarrhea, and burns.	Check urine output before infusing potassium. Continually assess for electrolyte or fluid imbalance: check laboratory values as well as signs and symptoms specific to imbalance. Assess for edema and crackles.
89 to 349 calories. Supplies calories as carbohydrates.	Do not infuse with blood. Assess patient for greater caloric need.
Both, 170 calories. For shock when blood products are not available. Increases blood volume, venous return, cardiac output; decreases blood viscosity and peripheral venous resistance; reduces aggregation of erythrocytes and other blood elements. Prophylaxis against venous thrombosis and thromboembolism inhibits vascular stasis and platelet adhesiveness. Priming solution for extracorporeal circulation.	Watch for allergic reactions (such as mild urticaria) and stop infusion immediately (these colloid hypertonic solutions attract water from the extravascular space and can cause fluid overload). Infuse cautiously in dehydrated patients, in whom additional fluid replacement will be needed. May prolong bleeding time and depress platelet function; may decrease renal and liver function. Can alter the following laboratory values: blood glucose, bilirubin, and total protein values; blood typing; cross matching; and tests with acids.
No calories. Test for renal function (oliguria from tubular necrosis). Diuretic therapy for intoxications, edema, and ascites.	Do not give to patients with impaired renal function who fail to respond to the test dose, with severe congestive heart failure, or with metabolic edema and head injuries. Low room temperature may cause crystallization. Use blood filter set to prevent infusion of mannitol crystals.

Appendix E

BLOOD COMPONENT THERAPY

All blood component products are extracted from whole blood, but because each has different characteristics, some components treat certain hematologic disorders better than others. The doctor will choose a blood component product based on how well it will treat your patient's condition. For example, if your patient needs volume replenishment quickly, he will receive a volume expander. If his blood is not clotting properly, he will receive a product with clotting factors. The table below reviews blood component products and their uses.

TYPE	CONTENTS	USES	NURSING CONSIDERATIONS
Whole blood	• Red blood cells (RBCs), white blood cells (WBCs), platelets, plasma, and plasma clotting factors	• To restore blood volume and to replenish oxygen-carrying capacity in a patient with massive hemorrhage	• Administer through a large-gauge needle or catheter over 2 to 4 hours, or as ordered.
Packed cells	• RBCs and 20% plasma • Less sodium and potassium than whole blood	• To replenish blood's oxygen-carrying capacity while minimizing risk of fluid overload in patients with severe anemia, slow blood loss, or congestive heart failure	• Administer more slowly than whole blood (unless diluted with normal saline solution).
Washed cells	• RBCs and 20% plasma • Fewer WBCs and platelets than packed cells	• To replenish blood's oxygen-carrying capacity in patients previously sensitized by transfusions	• Administer at a slower rate than whole blood (unless diluted with normal saline solution).
Granulocytes	• WBCs and 20% plasma	• To treat life-threatening granulocytopenia ($<500/mm^3$)	• Administer rapidly. • Expect the patient to develop fever, chills, hypertension, or disorientation during transfusion; these are considered transfusion reactions.

BLOOD COMPONENT THERAPY *(continued)*

TYPE	CONTENTS	USES	NURSING CONSIDERATIONS
Plasma (fresh frozen)	• Clotting factors II, III, V, VII, IX, X, and XIII; fibrinogen; prothrombin; albumin; and globulins	• To treat patients with clotting factor deficiencies (the only treatment for factor V deficiency) • To expand volume	• Fresh frozen plasma takes 20 minutes to thaw, so call the blood bank ahead of time. • Administer one unit over 1 hour.
Platelets	• Platelets, WBCs, and plasma	• To correct low platelet counts (<10,000/mm³)	• Administer one unit over 10 minutes.
Cryoprecipitate	• Factors VIII and XIII and fibrinogen	• To replace clotting factors in patients with disseminated intravascular coagulation, hemophilia A, von Willebrand's disease, fibrinogen deficiency, or factor XIII deficiency	• Administer rapidly immediately after thawing to ensure factor activation.
Albumin (5% and 25%)	• 5% and 25% albumin from plasma	• To replace volume in patients suffering from shock, burns, hypoproteinemia, or hypoalbuminemia	• Administer 1 ml/ minute or, if the patient is in shock, administer rapidly. • May administer with dextrose 5% in water.
Plasma protein fraction	• 5% albumin and globulin solution in normal saline solution	• To expand volume in patients with burns, hemorrhage, or hypoproteinemia	• Administer 1 ml/ minute. • Risk of hepatitis or sensitization is low.
Prothrombin	• Factors II, VII, IX, and X	• To replace clotting factors in patients with hemophilia B or bleeding secondary to severe liver disease	• Prothrombin is used infrequently because of increased hepatitis risk.

Index

t refers to a table.

t refers to a table.

Notes

Notes

Notes

Notes

Notes

Notes

Notes